Pain

Introducing Health Sciences: A Case Study Approach

Series editor: Basiro Davey

Seven case studies on major topics in global public health are the subject of this multidisciplinary series of books, each with its own animations, videos and learning activities on DVD. They focus on: access to clean water in an overcrowded and polluted world; the integration of psychological and biological approaches to pain; alcohol consumption and its effects on the body; the science, risks and benefits of mammography screening for early breast cancer; chronic lung disease due to smoke pollution – a forgotten cause of millions of deaths worldwide; traffic-related injuries, tissue repair and recovery; and the causes and consequences of visual impairment in developed and developing countries. Each topic integrates biology, chemistry, physics and psychology with health statistics and social studies to illuminate the causes of disease and disability, their impacts on individuals and societies and the science underlying common treatments. These case studies will be of value to anyone who is, or wants to be, working in a health-related occupation where scientific knowledge could enhance your prospects. If you have a wide-ranging interest in human sciences and want to learn more about global health issues and statistics, how the body works and the scientific rationale for screening procedures and treatments, this series is for you.

Titles in this series

Water and Health in an Overcrowded World, edited by Tim Halliday and Basiro Davey

Pain, edited by Frederick Toates

Alcohol and Human Health, edited by Lesley Smart

Screening for Breast Cancer, edited by Elizabeth Parvin

Chronic Obstructive Pulmonary Disease: A Forgotten Killer, edited by Carol Midgley

Trauma, Repair and Recovery, edited by James Phillips

Visual Impairment: A Global View, edited by Heather McLannahan

Pain

Edited by Frederick Toates

 The Open University

OXFORD
UNIVERSITY PRESS

Published by Oxford University Press, Great Clarendon Street, Oxford OX2 6DP
in association with The Open University, Walton Hall, Milton Keynes MK7 6AA.

Oxford University Press is a department of the University of Oxford. It furthers the University's
objective of excellence in research, scholarship, and education by publishing worldwide in

Oxford New York

Auckland Cape Town Dar es Salaam Hong Kong Karachi Kuala Lumpur Madrid Melbourne
Mexico City Nairobi New Delhi Shanghai Taipei Toronto

with offices in
Argentina Austria Brazil Chile Czech Republic France Greece Guatemala Hungary
Italy Japan Poland Portugal Singapore South Korea Switzerland
Thailand Turkey Ukraine Vietnam

Oxford is a registered trade mark of Oxford University Press in the UK and in certain
other countries.

Published in the United States by Oxford University Press Inc., New York

First published 2007

Edited, and designed by The Open University.

Typeset by SR Nova Pvt. Ltd, Bangalore India.

Printed and bound in the United Kingdom at the University Press, Cambridge.

This book forms part of the Open University course SDK125 *Introducing Health Sciences: A Case
Study Approach*. Details of this and other Open University courses can be obtained from the Student
Registration and Enquiry Service, The Open University, PO Box 197, Milton Keynes MK7 6BJ,
United Kingdom:
tel. +44 (0)870 333 4340, email general-enquiries@open.ac.uk.

http://www.open.ac.uk

British Library Cataloguing in Publication Data available on request

Library of Congress Cataloging in Publication Data available on request

ISBN 9780 1992 3736 4

10 9 8 7 6 5 4 3 2 1

ABOUT THIS BOOK

This book and the accompanying material on DVD present the second case study in a series of seven, under the collective title *Introducing Health Sciences: A Case Study Approach*. Together they form an Open University (OU) course for students beginning the first year of an undergraduate programme in Health Sciences. Each case study has also been designed to 'stand alone' for readers studying it in isolation from the rest of the course, either as part of an educational programme at another institution, or for general interest and self-directed study.

Pain is a multidisciplinary introduction to a topic of global importance for public health. This case study is for anyone seeking a scientific understanding of pain. In such a wide-ranging subject area, we have had to be selective, but we have included aspects of the biology, chemistry, psychology and epidemiology of the topic, as indicated in the contents list at the start of the book. No previous experience of studying science has been assumed and new concepts and specialist terminology are explained with examples and illustrations.

To help you plan your study of this material, we have included a number of 'icons' in the margin to indicate different types of activity which have been included to help you develop and practice particular skills. This icon indicates when to undertake an activity on the accompanying DVD. You will need to 'run' the DVD programs on your computer because they are *interactive*, and this function doesn't operate on a domestic DVD-player. The DVD presents four guided activities: the first gives an insight into the experience of chronic pain from the viewpoint of patients and staff at a pain treatment clinic; the second uses interactive animations to illustrate how the nervous system transmits signals, including those experienced as pain, and what happens at the synapse – the junction between neurons; the third introduces 'gate theory' – a unifying explanation of ways in which the experience of pain can be modified by signalling in the nervous system; the fourth activity explains some chemical, physiological and psychological treatments for chronic pain, when we revisit the pain clinics.

Activities involving pencil-and-paper exercises are indicated by this icon . One additional activity for Open University students only is described in a *Companion* text, which is not available outside the OU course. This is indicated by this icon in the margin. The reference to this activity for OU students is given in the margin of the book and should not interrupt your concentration if you are not studying it as part of an OU course.

At various points in the book, you will find 'boxed' material of two types: Explanation Boxes and Enrichment Boxes. The Explanation Boxes contain basic concepts explained in the kind of detail that someone who is completely new to the health sciences is likely to want. The Enrichment Boxes contain extension material, included for added interest, particularly if you already have some knowledge of basic science. If you are studying this book as part of an OU course, you should note that the Explanation Boxes contain material that is *essential* to your learning and which therefore may be *assessed*. However, the content of the Enrichment Boxes will *not* be tested in the course assessments. The authors' intention is to bring you into the subject, develop confidence through activities and guidance, and provide a stepping stone into further study. The most important terms appear in **bold** font in the text at the point where they are first defined, and these terms are also in bold in the index at the end of the book. Understanding of the meaning and uses of the bold terms is essential (i.e. assessable) if you are an OU student.

Active engagement with the material throughout this book is encouraged by numerous 'in text' questions, indicated by a diamond symbol (◆), followed immediately by our suggested answers. It is good practice always to cover the answer and attempt your own response to the question before reading ours. At the end of each chapter, there is a summary of the key points and a list of the main learning outcomes, followed by self-assessment questions to enable you to test your own learning. The answers to these questions are at the back of the book.

Internet database (ROUTES)

A large amount of valuable information is available via the internet. To help OU students and other readers of books in this series to access good quality sites without having to search for hours, the OU has developed a collection of internet resources on a searchable database called ROUTES. All websites included in the database are selected by academic staff or subject-specialist librarians. The content of each website is evaluated to ensure that it is accurate, well presented and regularly updated. A description is included for each of the resources.

The website address for ROUTES is: http://routes.open.ac.uk/

Entering the Open University course code 'SDK125' in the search box will retrieve all the resources that have been recommended for this book. Alternatively if you want to search for any resources on a particular subject, type in the words which best describe the subject you are interested in (for example, 'analgesia'), or browse the alphabetical list of subjects.

Authors' acknowledgements

As ever in The Open University, this book and DVD combine the efforts of many people with specialist skills and knowledge in different disciplines. The principal author was (text) Frederick Toates (psychology), who would like to acknowledge in particular the critical comments of Basiro Davey (public health), Bina Sharma (OU editor) and Paul Gabbott (biology). The DVD animations were written, devised and developed by Frederick Toates, with Brian Richardson (Science Web and Interactive Media team), Paul Gabbott and Steve Best (graphic artist). The audiovisual material was developed by Frederick Toates, Paul Gabbott, Hendrik Ball (independent producer) and Jo Mack (OU Sound and Vision).

Our contributions have been shaped and immeasurably enriched by the OU course team who helped us to plan the content and made numerous comments and suggestions for improvements as the material progressed through several drafts. It would be impossible to thank everyone personally, but we would like to acknowledge the help and support of academic colleagues who have contributed to this book (in alphabetical order of discipline): Nicolette Habgood, Heather

McLannahan, Carol Midgley and James Phillips (biology), Lesley Smart (chemistry), Jeanne Katz (health & social care), Elizabeth Parvin (physics) and Peter Naish (psychology).

We are very grateful to our External Assessor, Professor Susan Standring, Head of Department of Anatomy and Human Sciences, Kings College London, whose detailed comments have contributed to the structure and content of the book and kept the needs of our intended readership to the fore. We also acknowledge the valuable comments of our external critical reader, Dr Anthony Ordman (Royal Free Hospital, London).

Special thanks are due to all those involved in the OU production process, chief among them Joy Wilson and Dawn Partner, our wonderful Course Manager and Course Team Assistant, whose commitment, efficiency and unflagging good humour were at the heart of the endeavour. We also warmly acknowledge the contributions of Steve Best, our graphic artist, who developed and drew all the diagrams; Sarah Hofton, our graphic designer, who devised the page designs and layouts; and Martin Keeling, who carried out picture research and rights clearance. Activities to support Open University students in developing ICT skills and information literacy were devised by Dave Horan (iSkills Project), Clari Hunt (OU Library), Jamie Daniels (web developer) and Basiro Davey. The media project managers were Judith Pickering and James Davies.

For the copublication process, we would especially like to thank Jonathan Crowe of Oxford University Press and, from within The Open University, Christianne Bailey (Media Developer, Copublishing). As is the custom, any small errors or shortcomings that have slipped in (despite our collective best efforts) remain the responsibility of the authors. We would be pleased to receive feedback on the book (favourable or otherwise). Please write to the address below.

Dr Basiro Davey, SDK125 Course Team Chair

Department of Biological Sciences
The Open University
Walton Hall
Milton Keynes
MK7 6AA
United Kingdom

Environmental statement

Paper and board used in this publication is FSC certified.

Forestry Stewardship Council (FSC) is an independent certification, which certifies that the virgin pulp used to make the paper/board comes from traceable and sustainable sources from well-managed forests.

CONTENTS

1   PAIN: A GLOBAL HEALTH PROBLEM   1
Frederick Toates and Basiro Davey

1.1   A sensory and emotional experience   1

1.2   A psychobiological approach to pain   2

1.3   Measuring pain   2

Summary of Chapter 1   5

Learning outcomes for Chapter 1   6

Self-assessment questions for Chapter 1   6

2   DESCRIBING AND CLASSIFYING PAIN   7
Frederick Toates

2.1   The time factor   7

2.2   The range of uses of the term 'pain'   7

2.3   A fundamental distinction   10

Summary of Chapter 2   12

Learning outcomes for Chapter 2   13

Self-assessment questions for Chapter 2   13

3   HOW TO EXPLAIN PAIN: THE BASIC PRINCIPLES   15
Frederick Toates

3.1   Pain, evolution and the human zoo   15

3.2   The nature of pain   17

3.3   Interacting factors underlying pain   20

3.4   The link between stimuli and pain   21

3.5   Sociocultural, religious and gender factors   22

3.6   The role of the brain   22

3.7   The study of mind and consciousness   25

Summary of Chapter 3   28

Learning outcomes for Chapter 3   28

Self-assessment questions for Chapter 3   28

4	HOW THE BODY WORKS	31
	Frederick Toates	
4.1	Body systems	31
4.2	Cells	32
4.3	Homeostasis	34
4.4	The endocrine system	36
	Summary of Chapter 4	38
	Learning outcomes for Chapter 4	38
	Self-assessment questions for Chapter 4	38
5	THE NERVOUS SYSTEM	39
	Frederick Toates	
5.1	Nerves, neurons and axons	40
5.2	Types of neuron	40
5.3	The role of neurons	42
5.4	How do neurons perform their role?	44
5.5	Synapses	51
5.6	Some details of the brain	55
5.7	The somatic and autonomic nervous systems	58
	Summary of Chapter 5	60
	Learning outcomes for Chapter 5	61
	Self-assessment questions for Chapter 5	61
6	A FOCUS ON PAIN AND THE NERVOUS SYSTEM	63
	Frederick Toates	
6.1	The periphery	64
6.2	The spinal cord	66
6.3	The brain	68
6.4	Anomalies of pain	69
6.5	Relating nociceptive pain to psychogenic pain	73
	Summary of Chapter 6	74
	Learning outcomes for Chapter 6	75
	Self-assessment questions for Chapter 6	75

7	TREATING PAIN	77
	Frederick Toates	
7.1	Chemical interventions	77
7.2	Transcutaneous electrical nerve stimulation	81
7.3	Surgical intervention	82
7.4	Psychological intervention	82
	Summary of Chapter 7	85
	Learning outcomes for Chapter 7	86
	Self-assessment questions for Chapter 7	86
8	PLACEBO EFFECTS	89
	Frederick Toates	
8.1	Explaining the placebo effect	89
8.2	The psychobiology of the placebo effect	92
8.3	Implications of the placebo effect	92
	Summary of Chapter 8	93
	Learning outcomes for Chapter 8	93
	Self-assessment questions for Chapter 8	93
9	FINAL WORD	95
	Frederick Toates	
9.1	A challenging puzzle	95
9.2	Relevance of the meaning of 'psychological' and 'psychogenic'	97
9.3	Practical implications	97
	Summary of Chapter 9	98
	Learning outcomes for Chapter 9	98
	Self-assessment questions for Chapter 9	98
	ANSWERS AND COMMENTS	99
	REFERENCES AND FURTHER READING	103
	ACKNOWLEDGEMENTS	107
	INDEX	109

The DVD activities associated with this book were written, designed and developed by Hendrik Ball, Steve Best, Paul Gabbott, Jo Mack, Brian Richardson and Frederick Toates.

1 PAIN: A GLOBAL HEALTH PROBLEM

1.1 A sensory and emotional experience

This book examines a phenomenon that involves the body, behaviour and conscious mind: *pain*. Investigating how humans experience pain, what triggers it and why the experience can vary so greatly at different times is an enormous challenge. Consider some cases of pain (Vignette 1.1):

Vignette 1.1 Some cases of pain

- Helen is suffering from toothache. Until she felt the pain, Helen had no idea that anything was wrong with her teeth.

- Padmal is removing a thorn from his foot. He only knew of the thorn because of the pain.

- Ali has sprained his ankle while playing football and asks his friends to ease the pain by supporting him as he limps back to the team's changing room.

- Li Jun Ping has suffered a painful headache for several days. She has gone to a natural medicine clinic for massage treatment, which is more painful than the headache (Figure 1.1).

- Natasha is in hospital in continuous pain from a cancerous tumour. She obtains relief by means of injections of the powerful painkiller, morphine.

- Jack, a machine-operator, suffers from back pain. He has taken weeks off work and has plunged into deep depression.

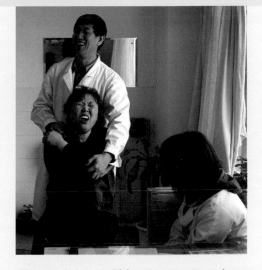

Figure 1.1 A Chinese woman endures a painful neck massage in a natural medicine clinic. What are the triggers to various types of pain? (Photo: Natalie Behring/Panos Pictures)

What do these six situations have in common? They all fit the definition of **pain** given by the International Association for the Study of Pain:

> An unpleasant sensory and emotional experience associated with actual or potential tissue damage, or described in terms of such damage.
>
> (IASP, 2007)

In each case, there is a physical disturbance in the body, which is the initial trigger to pain. In some cases, the disturbance is obvious, e.g. Padmal can see the thorn. In others, the disturbance might need specialised investigative techniques to reveal its nature.

Notice that the IASP definition refers to pain as a 'sensory *and* emotional experience'. However, such a definition does not enable you to predict how much distress would be felt by each of the six people described above. Pain is a **subjective experience**: that is to say, it is accessible only to the person who experiences it and pain is reported in terms of the sufferer's *inner* conscious 'mental world'. This is one of several difficulties for scientists investigating how pain arises and is felt. Another problem concerns the experimental study of pain. For obvious ethical and practical reasons, there are tight limits on the extent to which researchers can inflict pain.

1.2   A psychobiological approach to pain

This book adopts a **psychobiological approach** to understanding pain, which implies two closely related things. First, both the psychological and biological sciences have roles to play in understanding pain. Secondly, pain is a phenomenon that is *both* psychological and biological.

> Psychology is the scientific discipline engaged in the study of mind and behaviour. Biology is the study of the structure and functions of living organisms and their interactions in the natural world.

An example can help to illustrate what we mean by 'psychobiological'. Consider the phrase 'what's on your mind?' At the moment, your mind is (we assume!) focused on reading this book – your mind is 'processing information' presented as words. If you were to listen to the radio, your mind would be processing information on sounds. The basis of all such experiences of the *mind* is specific corresponding activity of the *brain*. By 'activity' is meant *electrical* activity: changes in such activity are the measure of the brain in action. The psychobiological approach defines the **mind** as being 'what the brain does': the mind *is* all the information-processing carried out by the brain.

> On the DVD that accompanies this book you will hear the expression that 'pain is a *biopsychosocial* phenomenon'. This means much the same thing as 'psychobiological' but also serves to draw attention to social interactions as part of the picture.

Thus, pain is simultaneously a psychological phenomenon, an experience of the conscious mind that includes how people perceive and interpret their pains – and a product of the body, a physical phenomenon. A physical disturbance in the body is communicated to the brain and this information is processed as pain. No matter where the disturbance arises, the fact that the mind is alerted to pain depends upon the physical structure of the brain.

Adopting a psychobiological approach, this book investigates some important questions in the scientific understanding of pain:

1   How can pain be described and classified (Chapter 2)?

2   How is information on a disturbance in the body (e.g. inflammation at the root of a tooth) conveyed to the brain, where it triggers pain? How do bodily events link to particular conscious experiences (Chapters 3 and 5)?

3   How does pain relate to the overall working of the body (Chapter 4)?

4   Are there specific parts of the brain that have a particular responsibility for the experience of pain (Chapters 3 and 6)?

5   How do therapeutic techniques work to counter pain (Chapter 7)?

6   How can certain puzzling features of pain be explained, such as the ability of a completely inert chemical to alleviate pain, or the 'phantom limb' pain felt after amputation (Chapters 6 and 8)?

1.3   Measuring pain

What is the extent of the role that pain plays in the lives of people around the world? How much distress and disability does it cause? The answer is that no-one knows precisely, but experts agree that pain is a major global health problem that tends to be neglected even in the richer nations.

◆ Why do you think statistics on the extent of pain are very difficult to collect, even in countries with well-organised disease registries?

◆ You might have thought of several reasons:

- Pain is a subjective experience; there is no objective test of whether someone is (or is not) in pain, or ways of measuring objectively 'how much' pain they are in.

- Pain might be intense but resolve swiftly (e.g. the pain of a cut finger), or persist for years (e.g. joint pain in arthritis), or 'come and go' (as in migraine headaches). It is difficult for data on pain to reflect such variations.

- Pain is associated with different diseases, disabilities and injuries; statistics may be collected on these conditions, rather than on the pain they cause (e.g. blocked arteries supplying the heart cause chest pain, but cases are recorded as *angina* not as examples of pain).

The term 'objective' means that something can be observed by more than one person and measured by agreed standards of measurement, as for height. By contrast, if something is 'subjective', it can only be described by the person who experiences it.

Reliable data are even harder to acquire in the world's poorer countries, where health statistics are not collected systematically. For all these reasons, estimating the frequency of pain across a population or between different countries is inherently problematic. Since researchers cannot measure pain directly, they resort to what are termed **proxy measures** of pain (a proxy 'acts on behalf of' or 'stands in' for something else). Thus, the extent of pain in a population can be estimated *indirectly* by measuring, for example, the number of days lost from work due to pain (e.g. Jack's back pain), or the number of prescriptions written for painkillers such as morphine (as in Natasha's case).

◆ Earlier we mentioned toothache, headache, cancer pain, back pain, arthritis, cuts and angina. What other diseases or states that are inherently painful could act as proxy measures for the burden of pain in a population?

◆ Conditions with a clear physical origin for the pain include childbirth; appendicitis; ear infections; broken bones and other injuries sustained in sports (such as Ali's sprained ankle), traffic accidents, falls, natural disasters, or those that follow violence.

Table 1.1 (overleaf) shows some global statistics to illustrate the ubiquity and variety of pain. Notice that over 313 million people were suffering from a migraine on the date this survey was carried out. Headaches are extraordinarily common sources of pain. The World Health Organization (WHO) estimates that over 60% of males and 80% of females in developed countries suffer 'tension type' headaches, and one adult in 20 has a headache every, or nearly every, day (WHO, 2004).

In Activity 3.1 on the DVD, Keelie exemplifies pain arising from physical violence while Naomi exemplifies it arising from a traffic accident.

Table 1.1 Worldwide incidence (number of new cases in a year) and prevalence (total number of cases in existence at the survey date) of selected painful conditions in 2002. (Source: data from WHO, 2002)

Incidence	World total
injuries due to traffic accidents	20 768 000
injuries due to interpersonal violence	16 115 000
self-inflicted injuries	10 170 000
Prevalence	
migraine	313 311 000
osteoarthritis	143 668 000
injured spinal cord	19 359 000

Note that the criteria determining eligibility to receive an incapacity benefit can change over time, and this will affect estimates of the extent of back pain based on this proxy measure.

Low back pain is the most common reason for days lost from work in industrialised societies such as the UK (Figure 1.2); between 59 and 85% of these populations will suffer back pain at some point in their lives (Andersson, 1999; Mounce, 2002). The causes include holding a standing posture for too long and mechanical strain due to heavy lifting or prolonged driving. Like Jack, many people with back pain also suffer from psychological distress such as depression. Occupational injuries to the back are even more common in developing countries, where workers are less well protected by health and safety practices (Figure 1.3).

A study in the USA found that, over a period of one year, roughly 70 million people (25% of the population) suffered acute, recurrent or chronic pain, and 10% experienced pain on at least 100 days a year (Gatchel and Weisberg, 2000). Such data are rarely obtained in developing countries, where scarce resources for data collection concentrate on infectious and chronic diseases.

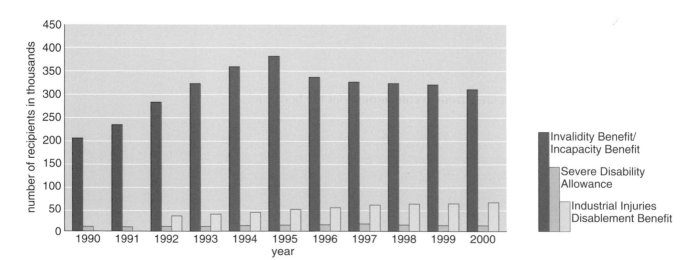

Figure 1.2 Bar chart showing the number of working-age recipients of social security benefits for incapacities of the back (in thousands) in the period 1990–2000 in the UK. (Source: data from Frank, 2002)

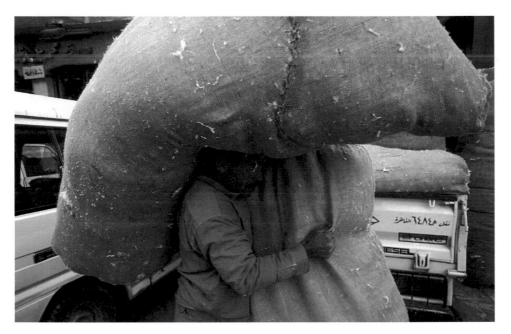

Figure 1.3   An Egyptian porter unloads bales of cotton. What kind of damage could this work be doing to his body? (Source: Mark Henley/Panos Pictures)

No-one suggests that there was a past 'golden age' in human evolution when pains were rare, but many of the sources of pain referred to in this chapter are a feature of the crowded, stressful urban environment (the 'human zoo') in which more than half of the world's population now live. For example, there were over 20 million injuries due to traffic accidents in 2002 (Table 1.1).

The next chapter will consider how to describe and classify pain, extending the range of pain-related situations from those introduced here.

Injuries due to traffic accidents are discussed in another book in this series *Trauma, Repair and Recovery* (Phillips, 2008).

Summary of Chapter 1

1.1   Pain commonly arises from a disturbance to the body, as in damage to a tissue.

1.2   A psychobiological approach to pain draws on both biology and psychology. Many pains arise from events throughout the body and information on them is conveyed to the brain. At the same time, pain is a feature of the conscious mind.

1.3   Pain is a major cause of suffering worldwide and an economic drain on individuals and nations through lost working hours.

1.4   Pain is a subjective experience, which means that it cannot be measured directly. Researchers have to employ 'proxy measures' of pain to estimate its extent.

Learning outcomes for Chapter I

After studying this chapter and its associated activities, you should be able to:

LO 1.1   Define and use, or recognise definitions and applications of, each of the terms printed in **bold** in the text. (Question 1.1)

LO 1.2   Describe what is meant by 'biological' and 'psychological' approaches to the study of pain and outline how a psychobiological approach draws from each perspective. (Question 1.1)

LO 1.3   Describe some of the problems in measuring pain and in estimating the burden of pain in populations. (Questions 1.2 and 1.3)

LO 1.4   Give examples to illustrate the extent of pain as a worldwide health problem. (Question 1.3)

Self-assessment questions for Chapter I

Question 1.1 (LOs 1.1 and 1.2)

How is a psychobiological approach to understanding the brain and mind relevant to the study of pain?

Question 1.2 (LO 1.3)

In what way is the study of pain more problematic than the study of (a) an infectious disease such as cholera or the common cold, or (b) the ability of your hand to reach out and grasp an object?

Question 1.3 (LOs 1.3 and 1.4)

Suggest a proxy measure that could be used to estimate the extent of minor, self-managed pain. What drawbacks do you foresee in interpreting the data you obtain?

2   DESCRIBING AND CLASSIFYING PAIN

Any scientific endeavour needs to build upon a system of description, definition and classification. Therefore, Chapter 2 will attempt to bring some initial clarity and order to the study of pain.

2.1   The time factor

A dimension along which pains can be classified is in terms of their duration (Sufka and Turner, 2005). However, somewhat confusingly, this classification also involves the nature of the trigger to the pain. What is termed **acute pain** lasts for only a relatively short time. It is associated with damage to a body region (e.g. a cut) and the duration of pain usually corresponds roughly to the continued existence of the disturbance to the body. Acute pains persuade people to act so as to escape the pain and later to protect the injured part until healing is completed. They also encourage people to avoid the pain-triggering situation in the future. In the case of surgical intervention or bone fracture, pain's duration often corresponds roughly with the time taken for healing (Cheville et al., 2000).

The expression **chronic pain** refers to pains that last from months to years. Chronic pain typically lasts long after the initial cause is corrected, e.g. long after the time required for healing following surgery to remove a tumour. Such pain becomes a medical problem in its own right and commonly triggers emotional disturbances such as depression.

2.2   The range of uses of the term 'pain'

What is the range of situations covered by the word 'pain'? A word can refer to a number of rather different things that all have something in common. For example, the word 'bird' describes things as different as eagles, ducks and wrens. Despite being very different, they have sufficient in common to make the single word 'bird' a useful one. So, consider the word 'pain' in terms of the examples that were used in Chapter 1. As was noted earlier, they are all instances of disturbances to the body that trigger an unpleasant state of mind that is labelled 'pain'.

So, by use of the term 'disturbance to the body', have we exhausted the range of situations associated with pain? The causes of some pains are only revealed, if at all, by sophisticated medical investigation. However, without any equipment or expertise, reflection can reveal a class of additional examples of where 'pain' is commonly employed.

◆   What is this class?

◆   Pain caused by emotional events.

Consider the following examples (Vignette 2.1):

> **Vignette 2.1   Some further examples of pain**
>
> - Parminder, a doctor in Kolkata, says that she is in great *pain* as a result of being jilted: 'It feels that my heart has been broken in two and the *hurt* feelings are unbearable. I am *cut* to the core and *scarred* for life'.
> - Ho, a student in Singapore, says that it *pains* him to see the suffering of humanity.
> - Irina, a single unemployed parent and victim of abuse, is in search of a fix of heroin, to ease the emotional *pain* of her existence in a run-down apartment in Moscow. Irina is aware of the risk of infection from shared needles but this does not deter her.

The 'pain' described in these three examples is obviously not triggered by damage to the body. However, people commonly use the expression in a way that suggests that such pain is similar to that caused by body injury. Is this just a case of a colourful and persuasive metaphor, not to be taken as a literal truth? You might be interested in the observation of the pop-star and campaigner, Bob Geldof, commenting on the end of a relationship of 19 years standing (cited by MacDonald and Leary, 2005):

> The physical pain alone was terrible. I always used to think the expression 'a broken heart' was just a metaphor. But it felt as if I was having a heart attack.

It is still controversial whether such 'emotional pain' should be put in the same class as the pain of, for example, a toothache. They are, of course, not identical conditions and they are not usually felt to be so. Given the somewhat speculative use of the term 'pain' to cover unpleasant emotional events, more traditional investigators might consider it safer to confine use of 'pain' to that associated with physical bodily injuries. It is in the nature of science that such controversy can arise and the discussion that is triggered forces investigators and therapists to think carefully about the issues and 'what is in a word'.

There are similarities between emotional pain and that triggered by physical injury. This book will show where the consideration of some overlap between them can provide insight. It can help the search to understand general characteristics of pain.

Such an approach dovetails with a development within pain research and therapy, which considers an important psychological contribution to a wide range of pains, no matter what their origin. Hence, even a pain such as that of cancer can be better understood by taking psychological factors into account (Sullivan, 2000).

Similarly, the psychological state of the individual is a factor in determining the magnitude of low back pain (Mounce, 2002). A given degree of degenerative change of the spine, as revealed by an X-ray, can be associated with intense pain in one individual but no pain in another. People with low back pain often report more distress than can be accounted for by an objective assessment of their physical condition (Phillips and Gatchel, 2000). Psychological differences between different individuals are one possible explanatory factor here.

Of course, use of the term 'psychological factors' should in no way be used to undermine the 'real' nature of the pain. Now attempt Activity 2.1.

Activity 2.1 Types of pain

Allow about 10–15 minutes

Take another look at the examples of 'pain' in Vignettes 1.1 and 2.1 and try to recall some in your own personal experience. Then consider the following questions:

(i)   What is common in all the experiences described by the term 'pain'?

(ii)   Are there sufficient common features to justify the use of the single term 'pain'?

(iii) Are there fundamentally different types of pain that are collected together under the same heading?

(iv)   If you were to meet someone who claimed never to have experienced pain, how would you describe it to them?

Comments

The answers to these four questions might well run along the following lines.

(i)   Pain, of whatever form, takes command of attention and the conscious mind. It is difficult, if not impossible, to ignore pain. All pains are signals that cause us to take the action that appears to be appropriate to lowering the pain, e.g. removing a thorn, contacting the dentist, seeking support when walking on an injured limb or looking for drugs to lift emotional pain. In many cases, there is the opportunity to learn to avoid the pain in the future by altering behaviour, e.g. to wear shoes so as to avoid thorns or to drink less alcohol to avoid a hangover. What does Parminder's pain at being jilted motivate her to do? The possibilities include desperate emails and phone calls to try to restore the lost love, to seeking solace with family, to taking alcohol, or even, in the extreme and mercifully rare cases, to murder or suicide. So, each pain motivates the sufferer to take action such as to try to lower the pain. As another example, people commonly use the term 'pain' to refer to empathy for the suffering of another person, as in 'I feel your pain with you. I know what you are going through'. This often motivates giving to charity or offers of help for people who are sick, bereaved or going through an emotional crisis.

(ii)   Those common features listed under answer (i) would appear to justify trying to apply a single term to all such instances.

(iii) As a first approximation, 'pain' is used to refer to *either* a result of damage to the body *or* the result of certain emotional events. However, such a clear distinction can sometimes be misleading since the pains arising from bodily damage are affected by emotional events.

(iv) You would have great difficulty in conveying this inner subjective feeling of pain to someone who claimed never to have experienced it. You might try establishing a scale of the person's likes and dislikes and then locate pain on the extreme negative end of this. Also, you might try explaining in terms of the types of behaviour that pain triggers and the body's internal reactions, e.g. heart-rate acceleration, though, of course, this would not capture the emotive essence of the subjective aspect.

The principal concern in this book will be with pain arising from damage to the body but we will also give some consideration to emotional pain and empathy.

2.3   A fundamental distinction

In the case of such things as toothache and muscle pain, there is clearly an identifiable site of damage to tissue in the body and this is often the initial trigger to pain. For cancer, there is often a measurable disturbance to tissue at one or more sites. Such sites of disruption can be objectively located by a surgeon, doctor or dentist, and often a layperson. For sufferer and professional, the trigger to pain has a point of reference.

Such things as cuts and swellings, i.e. localisable triggers to pain involving tissue damage and which arise at the skin or within the body, are termed **noxious stimuli**. These stimuli can be defined by their physical and chemical properties, such as excessive cold or heat, swelling, acidity and cuts to the skin, etc. Derived from the same root as 'noxious', the process of detecting physically damaging stimuli by the body is termed **nociception** (pronounced roughly as noh-see-sep-shun). Pain triggered in this way is sometimes termed **nociceptive pain** in reference to the noxious stimulus.

So far, so good then, but, as will be discussed throughout the book, there is a complication. Some might term this the 'paradox of pain' (Melzack and Wall, 1988) and it is contained within the following combination of two observations:

*   An initial trigger to pain in the form of physical damage in the body, a noxious stimulus, can very often be identified.
*   Sometimes, the intensity of pain *bears little relation to the extent of the damage.*

Various factors in addition to tissue damage, e.g. psychological stress, will often also play an important part in pain. In other words, the input to the brain from the signal of damage in the body is *only one* of numerous determinants of pain. The brain is never inactive, even in sleep. Any nociceptive input arriving at the brain is set against the pattern of activity in the brain at that time. Expressed in terms of thought processes, the input is placed into a context of meaning and interpretation by the brain. These are fundamental principles for understanding pain and cautions to keep in mind throughout.

By contrast to noxious stimuli, the pain of social rejection or empathy for another's suffering obviously does not relate to a noxious stimulus in one's body. Rather, it arises from a complex *interpretation* by the brain of the social links between people or an ability to imagine the suffering mind of another (Figure 2.1). Psychologists employ the term **psychogenic stimuli** for the triggers to pain that *arise* from psychological causes such as loss and rejection. Such pain is termed **psychogenic pain.**

You might be tempted to refer to the pain triggered by psychogenic stimuli as 'psychological pain' but you would need to be very cautious. In keeping with a psychobiological approach, the pain is still *simultaneously* biological, since it arises in the brain. In order to undermine the temptation to create a rigid and clear-cut distinction between types of pain that are *either* biological *or* psychological, consider the following complications:

(i)   In seeking heroin to relieve social distress, Irina describes her pain as 'emotional' and therefore the temptation might be to classify it as 'psychological'. However, Irina's solution is to seek a *chemical* cure. Heroin has identifiable effects on the body. It is a substance with almost identical effects to morphine, which is used to treat serious nociceptive pain. Similarly, Parminder might seek solace in alcohol, which is a chemical having known effects on the physical body.

The effects of alcohol are described in another book in this series *Alcohol and Human Health* (Smart, 2007).

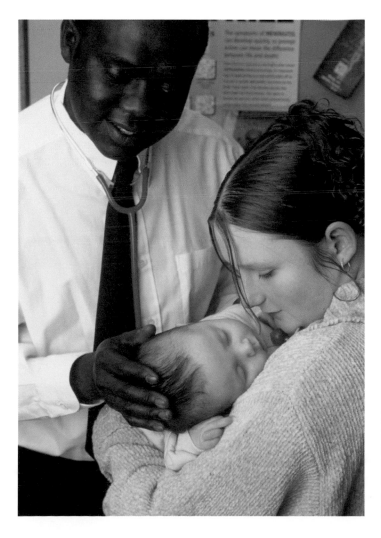

Figure 2.1   Human concern for another sentient being is easily recognised and generally regarded as a noble aspect of our make-up. Can science say anything about it? (Photo: Science Photo Library)

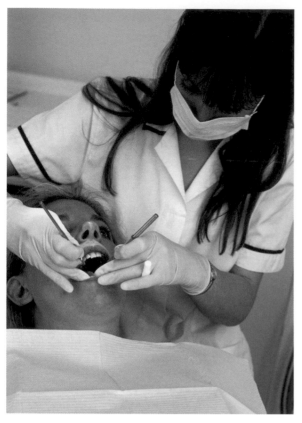

Figure 2.2 How does the dentist know that Helen is in pain? (Photo: Francois Sauze/Science Photo Library)

(ii) Helen has a toothache, which one might be tempted to call 'non-psychological' or 'physical'. Indeed, the rot at the root of her tooth and the swelling are unambiguously physical disturbances. The rotting tooth sets up increased activity in 'pain regions' of Helen's brain. Yet, an account just in terms of such physical events, though entirely valid and essential to understanding pain, misses out something fundamental. Our assumption that Helen is in pain is based primarily upon *her* report of a bad subjective experience, which, of course, cannot be observed directly (Figure 2.2). Helen's *mind* is dominated with the pain of her toothache. So, in one sense of the word, Helen's experience also sounds 'psychological'. Indeed, it appears that the amount of suffering will depend not only on the swelling but also on Helen's personality and culture, etc.

(iii) Natasha is in chronic pain, treated by morphine. In one study some years ago, very occasionally, as a test for how effective morphine is, patients were given an injection that contained no morphine at all. However, they were led to *believe* that it was morphine and they obtained pain relief all the same (Beecher, 1959; Melzack and Wall, 1988). A belief sounds to be something psychological and yet it affects the sensation of pain triggered by physical causes in the body.

(iv) Relief of nociceptive pain can sometimes be produced by psychological therapies such as distraction, meditation, hypnosis and learning to place a more positive interpretation on the situation. Conversely, if the patient places a catastrophic interpretation on the pain (e.g. 'the pain will surely kill me'), this can make it feel worse.

(v) Sometimes 'physical' pain is experienced as arising in a part of the body but no damage can be found that is triggering it (Cheville et al., 2000). Psychological factors can powerfully influence such pain.

(vi) People with a high tendency to suffer from depression also have a high tendency to experience chronic pain (Roth, 2000). The outlook for low back pain is worse if the patient shows depression, is unemployed or has a history of sexual abuse (Mounce, 2002). The existence of prior psychological distress such as anxiety is a factor that increases the probability of back pain arising (Andersson, 1999). That is to say, psychogenic factors can exacerbate nociceptive pain.

(vii) Finally, there is a result that emerged in 2003, with the development of technical equipment to generate images of brain activity, so-called 'imaging techniques' (Eisenberger et al., 2003). Researchers had already identified a collection of different regions of the brain, termed the **pain matrix**, which exhibits a relatively high activity at times of nociceptively triggered pain. It was found that some of these same regions are also activated at times of psychogenically triggered pain of social rejection. This result is potentially of enormous importance to our understanding of pain, emotion and distress, as well as the 'human condition' in the most fundamental sense. It will be discussed further in Chapter 6.

Summary of Chapter 2

2.1   The term 'pain' is used primarily to describe 'nociceptive pain', which arises from a disturbance by a noxious stimulus to a site in the body.

2.2   As a less traditional use of the term 'pain', 'psychogenic pain' is said to arise from psychogenic triggers, such as social loss.

2.3   Pain of any kind commands attention and is a signal to take action so as to lower the level of pain.

2.4   Nociceptive pains can often be influenced by a range of psychological factors, such as hope and despair.

2.5   All pains are simultaneously physical (involving the brain and, for nociceptive pain, the body outside the brain) and psychological. All pains occupy the conscious mind.

Learning outcomes for Chapter 2

After studying this chapter and its associated activities, you should be able to:

LO 2.1   Define and use, or recognise definitions and applications of, each of the terms printed in **bold** in the text. (Questions 2.1 and 2.2)

LO 2.2   Describe a range of situations that are associated with use of the term 'pain' and what they have in common, while distinguishing between nociceptive and psychogenic triggers to pain. (Questions 2.1 and 2.2)

LO 2.3   Explain why the term 'psychogenic pain' is preferred to 'psychological pain' and describe what misunderstanding could arise from use of the latter term. (Questions 2.1 and 2.2)

Self-assessment questions for Chapter 2

Question 2.1 (LOs 2.1, 2.2 and 2.3)

With regard to nociceptive pain, the chapter claimed that '…sometimes, the intensity of pain that is experienced *bears little relation to the extent of the damage*'. In what way does the study of psychological distress support this claim?

Question 2.2 (LOs 2.1, 2.2 and 2.3)

How has the use of brain imaging techniques provided insight into psychogenic pain?

3 HOW TO EXPLAIN PAIN: THE BASIC PRINCIPLES

Chapters 1 and 2 described the nature of pain and how to classify it. They suggested the need for psychological and biological perspectives to be brought to the explanation of pain. Chapter 3 looks in more detail at what is involved in these perspectives and how to describe and explain pain in subjective and objective terms. We examine how biological and psychological insights can be gained and the understanding to be derived from cross-cultural perspectives. First, we turn to a consideration of evolution and the 'human zoo'.

3.1 Pain, evolution and the human zoo

It is easy to appreciate the benefit of a number of pains, which are triggered by damage or potential damage to the body. Obviously, damage to body tissues is threatening to the workings of the body. Folk wisdom reinforces the intuitive notion that, for example, you need to get a thorn out of the foot or rest a strained muscle. Otherwise, the damage is likely to get worse. In a case such as a cut on the foot, there is a risk of infection and, as a result, even loss of part of the body. Similarly, putting extra strain on a muscle that is already disrupted can only make matters worse. By taking appropriate action, people are able to minimise the damage. Pains tend to cause people to limit their mobility and this aids the process of healing any damage to the body. Similarly, by resting in response to the bodily pains of an infection, people tend to speed their recovery. Common sense informs us in this way and medical science can put this on a more formal footing. In addition, this understanding can be reinforced by a consideration of some principles of evolution. These principles also help to make sense of what might otherwise be some puzzling features of pain.

3.1.1 The adaptive value of pain

Viewed in terms of evolution, the general principle of taking appropriate action to lower pain can be understood in terms of pain's **adaptive value**. If characteristics have served to increase the survival and reproductive chances of the animal (human or otherwise), such characteristics are said to have 'adaptive value'. For example, a capacity to feel pain and to react to it has adaptive value, since animals with this capacity have tended to avoid harm. It appears that some of the pains that humans experience today can be understood rather straightforwardly in such terms.

◆ Try to speculate on some instances of pain that arise from causes that were probably equally present in our early evolutionary environment as they are now and which reflect the adaptive value of pain.

◆ Pains arising from cuts, bruises, fractures, excesses of heat and cold and strains to muscles are probably equally represented in each situation. Such pains might seem to be the inevitable outcome of damage that arises when interacting with any environment. Similarly, the cramping pain from holding a fixed body position for too long would probably be present throughout human evolution.

Another book in this series *Water and Health in an Overcrowded World* (Halliday and Davey, 2007) introduces evolution, adaptation, evolutionary trade-off and the 'human zoo'.

◆ What are some examples of the actions that humans take to alleviate pain that are likely to have been equally present in the early environment of human evolution?

◆ Such things as protecting a damaged limb, attempting to remove a thorn from the foot and resting in response to pain were doubtless always around. (You might have noticed injured pets such as cats or dogs showing such reactions. Immobility in response to the pain of an infection has a wide representation throughout different species.)

◆ Suggest some actions to alleviate pain that involve modern inventions.

◆ These include the use of tablets and the hypodermic syringe to administer painkilling drugs.

Also pointing to pain's usefulness, occasionally people are born insensitive to pain and suffer repeated injuries to their bodies from burning, bone damage, infections at the site of injury and holding a fixed body position for too long. They rarely survive beyond their twenties (Sufka and Turner, 2005).

One can equally see the experience of pain in response to a broken social bond as serving an adaptive role. Social bonds, with their powerful emotional associations, were important for maintaining human survival chances in their evolutionary past and perpetuating genes when mates were found and children reared. Humans are social group-living animals, whose survival has surely depended on cooperation and mutual defence. Groups are held together by ties of kinship, friendship and interdependency. There would appear to be a strong adaptive value for a process which guarantees that any threats to a social bond tend to trigger action to oppose the threat. For the young mammal, social loss could herald a death sentence as surely as serious physical injury. A part of what keeps social bonds together appears to be the pain that arises from their breaking or threats that this might happen. Painful empathy for the suffering of a close relative or tribal member will tend to motivate caring activities.

In a range of other situations, what appears to have had adaptive value in the early evolutionary environment can now (in the modern 'human zoo') tend to produce behaviour that is to the detriment of survival. The expression 'human zoo' refers to the fact that very many humans now live in large urban environments that are very different from that of early human evolution. In this regard, such humans can be compared with animals living in a zoo.

For example, a fondness for sweet tastes was surely adaptive when the ancestors of modern humans were foraging for rare fruits. These days, in the 'human zoo' of affluent Western countries, there is an abundance of energy-rich sweet foods, located no further than a short drive away to the supermarket. In this environment, the characteristic that was once adaptive is something of a mixed blessing, as evidenced by the current epidemic of obesity. Similarly, it was of adaptive value to have processes that poured the hormone epinephrine into the bloodstream and thereby accelerated heart rate on confrontation with dangerous wild animals or enemies. One can speculate that such processes are still useful in sudden emergencies such as running from danger. However, these days, the same

◆ _____

Epinephrine was formerly known as adrenalin; you will still find the older term used in some textbooks and in everyday speech.

processes can work in 'over-drive' day-after-day, for example in people stuck in traffic jams and in competitive stress-inducing occupations. Such activation appears to serve little or no value and can be to the detriment of health.

3.1.2   Chronic pain as an evolutionary trade-off

There are instances of pain observed these days which might appear to be mysterious until viewed in terms of adaptation to an earlier environment. For example, Natasha's pain from cancer is utterly debilitating and appears to be doing little or nothing to help her recovery. It has become a major part of the *problem* rather than a part of the *solution*. Similarly, these days the pain of arthritis takes a terrible toll in terms of human mobility and well-being. So, such continuous pain might at first appear to make little sense when considering adaptive value. However, in terms of an **evolutionary trade-off**, it is necessary to consider that the processes underlying pain were 'good enough' for the problems confronted in the early environment. If pain were 'tuned' to be any less intense, our ancestors might have failed to respect it sufficiently. If it were more intense, it could cause more restraint than is justified.

Life expectancy was much less in those days. Much chronic pain in contemporary society is a feature of advanced years, beyond the age when reproduction would normally have occurred. Hence, we can speculate that such pain would have had little role in influencing the direction of human evolution.

3.2   The nature of pain

As noted earlier, pain is a *subjective experience*. Herein, a problem lies: science traditionally deals with *objective data*, things that can be *measured* precisely such as height or body temperature. This is 'public data', available to anyone with measuring equipment and willing participants. One scientist's measurement can be checked by another and the data recorded objectively, for example, on a graph. Such measurement does not depend upon a statement by the participants of their inner subjective experience.

Even given its subjective nature, is it still possible to *measure* pain, albeit in an unusual sense of the term 'to measure'? Researchers and therapists can ask participants to rate their pain on a scale of intensity ranging from zero, through mild (say 5 units) to very severe (say, 100 units). Participants or patients can be requested to describe the pain's quality, such as burning or itching. This, of course, yields a rather different kind of measurement from that of objective science.

◆ In what sense is it different?

◆ Being subjective, the results are unique to that individual at that moment in time and cannot be verified independently by anyone else.

Table 3.1 (overleaf) shows the result of research into the language used by people to describe their pains. Six different types of pain were associated with particular words and this has proved successful in helping to communicate information that is clinically relevant. Patients described different dimensions of the experience.

Table 3.1 Patients' descriptions of their pains. N = the number of participants in the study. (Source: Melzack and Wall, 1988, p. 42)

Menstrual pain ($N = 25$)	Arthritic pain ($N = 16$)	Labour pain ($N = 11$)	Disc disease pain ($N = 10$)	Toothache ($N = 10$)	Cancer pain ($N = 8$)
Sensory					
cramping (44%)	gnawing (38%)	pounding (37%)	throbbing (40%)	throbbing (50%)	shooting (50%)
aching (44%)	aching (50%)	shooting (46%)	shooting (50%)	boring (40%)	sharp (50%)
		stabbing (37%)	stabbing (40%)	sharp (50%)	gnawing (50%)
		sharp (64%)	sharp (60%)		burning (50%)
		cramping (82%)	cramping (40%)		heavy (50%)
		aching (46%)	aching (40%)		
			heavy (40%)		
			tender (50%)		
Affective					
tiring (44%)	exhausting (50%)	tiring (37%)	tiring (46%)	sickening (40%)	exhausting (50%)
sickening (50%)		exhausting (46%)	exhausting (40%)		
		fearful (36%)			
Evaluative					
	annoying (38%)	intense (46%)	unbearable (40%)	annoying (50%)	unbearable (50%)
Temporal					
constant (56%)	constant (44%)	rhythmic (91%)	constant (80%)	constant (60%)	constant (100%)
	rhythmic (56%)		rhythmic (70%)	rhythmic (40%)	rhythmic (88%)

The *sensory* dimension describes the quality of the pain in terms of the kind of event that would normally trigger such a sensation. The *affective* dimension describes the kind of feelings that the pain triggered. The term *evaluative* is used to estimate the intensity of the pain. The dimension *temporal* describes the length of time over which the pain is present and its pattern over time. Furthermore, following a particular injury, the nature of the pain can change over time, as healing progresses and inflammation subsides.

Wound healing is the topic of another book in this series (Phillips, 2008).

One study (Dubuisson and Melzack, 1976) showed that, on the basis of the words chosen by patients with eight different painful conditions, a computer was able to identify correctly the cause of pain in 77% of cases. When the sex of the patients and the location of pain were included, all of the cases were correctly diagnosed. So, the subjective report of the patient is an invaluable diagnostic aid.

For very young children or for people whose language capacities have been impaired, another scale can be used (Wong et al., 2001). Patients can point to the face that most accurately reflects their level of suffering (Figure 3.1).

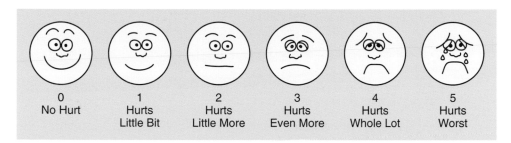

| 0 | 1 | 2 | 3 | 4 | 5 |
| No Hurt | Hurts Little Bit | Hurts Little More | Hurts Even More | Hurts Whole Lot | Hurts Worst |

Figure 3.1 The Wong–Baker Faces pain scale. (Source: Wong et al., 2001, Table 21-2, p. 691)

In some cases, observers can identify and even measure the causes of pain in the body that trigger the subjective experience, such as a thorn or a tumour. Investigators can also observe objective reactions associated with pain. These are both internal, such as changes in heart rate (number of beats per minute) and activity of the brain, and external, such as writhing and wincing. Finally, researchers and therapists try to link the subjective and objective evidence, in understanding a person's pain. Now attempt Activity 3.1.

Activity 3.1 Patients' experiences of pain

Allow 30 minutes for this activity

Now would be an ideal time to study the video entitled 'Patients' experiences of pain' which you will find on the DVD associated with this book. Patients at a pain clinic describe their experiences of pain and some of the treatments that they receive. If you are unable to study this video now, continue with the rest of the chapter and return to it as soon as you can.

Note the use of the term 'analgesics' in the video. It is explained later in the book but for now it is sufficient to know that it refers to a class of chemical used to reduce pain.

On watching this sequence, you are asked to observe carefully how patients describe their pains, in terms of the pains' quality, duration and location. Note the kind of terms that they employ. Note also how some patients make use of comparisons with familiar situations ('metaphors') to try to get across how the pain feels (e.g. 'it felt just like…'). When you have watched the video, try the following questions:

(i)   What kind of expressions were used?

(ii)   Compare the terms employed by the patients in the video with those of Table 3.1.

Comment

(i) *Brian* described his pain as 'dull aching', in terms of its quality. He used the term 'constant' to describe pain in the dimension of time. He employed the term 'in my stump' to describe its location. In terms of a comparison with the familiar, Brian used the expression 'electric shocks, which pulsate'.

Jo described her pain with the terms 'stabbing', 'crushing' and 'grinding'. In terms of location she described the 'spine' and, for duration, she used the term '24/7'. As a metaphor, she used the expressions 'someone grinding with their knuckles all day long' and 'electric volt'.

Keelie described her pain in terms of the 'base of my back' and 'spine' as its location', leaving parts of her body 'numb'.

David described the 'neck', 'arm', 'tips of fingers' and 'chest' as the bodily locations associated with the pain'.

(ii) You will see some overlap in the terms used by patients, but also that patients bring their own rich and personalised ways of describing their pain.

3.3 Interacting factors underlying pain

So far, we have distinguished between two broad categories of trigger to pain (nociceptive and psychogenic) and considered common features in the experience of pain caused by these triggers. As noted, there can be interaction between these triggers. The notions of 'common features' and 'interaction' are compatible with a number of phenomena, as follows (MacDonald and Leary, 2005):

1 Individuals who are described as 'introverts' (i.e. those usually wishing to avoid excessive social stimulation) tend to show a higher level of reaction to both nociceptive and psychogenic triggers to pain than do those classified as 'extroverts' (i.e. those who seek relatively more social stimulation).

2 Social support tends to reduce the intensity of both types of pain, whereas social conflict tends to exacerbate both.

3 Individuals who are particularly sensitive to hurt feelings also find noxious stimuli particularly painful.

4 Individuals having a strong fear of social abandonment tend to experience nociceptive triggers to pain as more distressing than secure individuals do. For people who are prone to anxiety and depression, there is a high tendency to experience pain that is excessive relative to the objective magnitude of the trigger (Gatchel and Weisberg, 2000).

5 Pain triggered by either nociceptive or psychogenic triggers increases the tendency to suffer depression and to display crying and aggression.

6 Pain is sometimes perceived in terms of noxious stimuli yet it is impossible to find a noxious stimulus that is triggering it. This is termed 'somatisation' or 'somatisation disorder'. An example is pain that appears to be very much like angina, a condition which is associated with the heart. However, no abnormality of the heart can be found. Pain occurs over long periods and

The term 'somatisation' derives from the Greek word 'soma', meaning 'the body'.

can sometimes be helped by psychological interventions. Stress, anxiety and depression commonly accompany and exacerbate the condition (Looper and Kirmayer, 2002).

Trying to tease apart exactly 'what causes what' can be difficult in the study of humans. For example, the evidence suggests that depression contributes to pain.

◆ Why must investigators be careful in drawing such a conclusion?

◆ A correlation between depression and pain does not prove a causal connection. In addition to depression contributing to pain, the experience of pain doubtless contributes to depression. Both could be associated independently with some other factor (e.g. worry about unemployment).

Later in the chapter, we will consider further evidence pointing to common features and the interaction between types of trigger to pain, after details of the brain have been described.

3.4   The link between stimuli and pain

We noted earlier a paradox in the study of pain and it will form a central feature throughout this book, as we attempt to unravel its basis. It is worth repeating the paradox, as follows.

Researchers can identify a range of noxious stimuli that *normally* trigger pain and they can link such stimuli with activity in particular brain regions. They can also document the qualities and intensity of pain that patients associate with these triggers. However, there is not always a close association between the actual amount of pain felt and what might objectively appear to be the trigger. Sometimes there can be damage with little experience of pain and conversely there can be serious pain of apparent nociceptive origin with little evidence of a noxious stimulus. There are several examples that illustrate this.

One case was documented in World War II. American soldiers, who were evacuated from battlefields while suffering very serious injuries, reported rather little pain (Beecher, 1946). This was attributed to their psychological state being one of honourable escape. Only on reaching hospital, did their pain become evident. It seems that pain is inhibited at times when it would not be in the individual's interest to be distracted. Rather, determination in the face of injury is the appropriate strategy (Figure 3.2).

People tend to assume that severe pain arising from, say, an arthritic knee implies a severe level of disease but this is not always so (Keefe et al., 2005). Similarly, an intuitive assumption is that, if pain arises from a malignant tumour, removing the tumour will remove the pain, but this is not invariably so.

Such evidence reinforces the conclusion that pain cannot be understood simply as a straightforward ('one-to-one') reaction to noxious stimuli. It is under the control of multiple factors, only

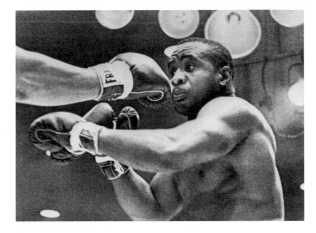

Figure 3.2   The American boxer Sonny Liston was once reported to have carried on a fight even with a broken jaw. Under what circumstances does tissue injury have relatively little effect? (Photo: Topham)

one of which is any noxious stimulus. That is to say, the capacity of a noxious stimulus to trigger pain depends also on the *context* in which it occurs. Such observations are crucial in developing a psychobiological account of pain.

In trying to understand pain, it can be useful to distinguish between its different features (Wade and Price, 2000). One is the *threshold*, the intensity of noxious stimulation at which a person first reports the sensation of pain. Another is the unpleasantness rating of the pain. The third is the emotional suffering and finally there is pain-related behaviour. The next section addresses these distinctions.

3.5   Sociocultural, religious and gender factors

Comparing across groups of people, how pains are expressed can show considerable variation. For example, Americans appear to be more disrupted behaviourally and professionally by back-pain arising from a particular intensity of stimulus than do Japanese (Hobara, 2005). One survey of the area (Edwards et al., 2001, p. 135) came to the tentative conclusion that African-Americans and white-Americans might '…differ in their responses to and tolerance of experimentally induced pain'. The authors add that any such differences might reflect different lifetime stress levels between ethnic groups. Of course, any differences between ethnic groups should not detract from the large differences within a given group.

Do differences between ethnic groups mean that the group *expressing* pain more is actually *suffering* more pain than the less-expressive group? In a study in Kuwait, it was found that, compared with Kuwaiti and Palestinian mothers, Bedouin mothers exhibited remarkably little pain-related behaviour at childbirth (Harrison, 1991). Yet, on a pain-rating scale, the groups of women gave their ratings as being roughly the same. Thus an absence of outward expression of pain cannot be assumed to reflect an absence of suffering.

Differences in the *meaning* attributed to pain can also play a role in how it is expressed. Some people of religious faith or who follow a Buddhist philosophy accept pain as an inevitable part of life or even a means to spiritual growth. Others, with no such convictions, might tend to see it simply as an unmitigated evil (McLachlan and Waldenström, 2005). The pain of childbirth is one that accompanies an act of great meaning for many women and its significance might help in coping with the pain (Callister et al., 1999).

To some extent the expression of pain depends upon cultural expectations and norms. In a number of cultures, it is more accepted as a 'cultural norm' for women to express pain than it is for men to do so (Hobara, 2005).

3.6   The role of the brain

3.6.1 Evidence for the role

In the study of conscious sensations such as joy, pain or grief, the brain forms a central part of the description and explanation. As noted earlier, the brain is assumed to be at the basis of what is called the 'mind' and it is not difficult to appreciate the central importance of the brain for the experience of pain. However, there is a tendency simply to take for granted that the brain is at the basis of mental life, so it is useful to be reminded of the evidence for this assumption. This includes:

- In Alzheimer's disease, identifiable degeneration of the brain is associated with loss of mental capacities, as in failures of memory and attention.

- Damage to particular brain regions is followed by particular types of disruption, for example, loss of hearing or vision.

- Under anaesthetic, conscious awareness of events is lost, together with pain. Anaesthetic applied to a part of the brain is followed by a loss of mental activities associated with that part.

- Drugs such as alcohol affect the brain and thereby alter mental activity.

Specifically, concerning pain, evidence of the involvement of the brain includes:

- With the help of modern technology, specific parts of the brain can be observed to change their activity when a noxious stimulus is applied to a part of the body.

- Surgical removal of particular parts of the brain can lower pain.

- Hypnosis can sometimes lower pain and this is associated with a change in activity in the brain.

- After a limb is lost, pain that appears to be coming from the missing limb is sometimes still felt. The pain is associated with activity of the brain's pain-related regions.

So, in general terms, an issue to be considered is – how is information on light, sound and touch, etc. communicated to the brain, so as to produce conscious sensations? More specifically, given the topic of this book, how do disturbances to the body in the form of, for example, cuts and bruises, communicate with the brain so as to produce the conscious sensation of pain?

3.6.2 The brain and its links with the body

All information, whether from the eyes, ears, nose, or tongue or touch, or from disturbances to the body as in noxious stimuli, is communicated to the brain via specialised structures ('communication channels') that are termed **nerves** (we will go into the details concerning nerves later). Figure 3.3 shows some nerves in relation to the brain and the **spinal cord**. The spinal cord is housed in the backbone and is a central channel for information passing between the brain and the parts of the body below the neck. Note some of the nerves of the body (coloured green). Such nerves convey information *to* the spinal cord and also convey information *from* the spinal cord. For example, information conveyed to the spinal cord concerns events such as tissue damage in the periphery of the body. Information coming from the spinal cord causes muscles to contract and thereby movement to occur.

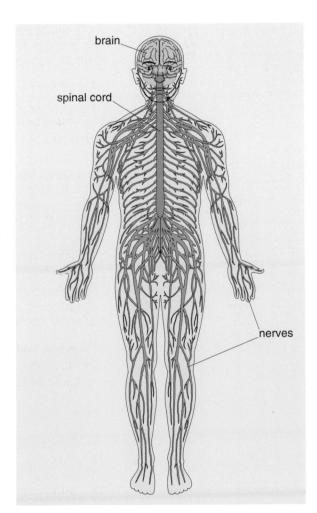

Figure 3.3   The body showing its nerves, the brain and spinal cord.

Information linking the brain and the body below the neck travels to and from the brain via the spinal cord. Above the neck, nerves pass directly between the brain and the head outside the brain.

Everyday language contains at least a small grain of truth, in that nerves are assumed to be involved with activities of a psychological nature. Expressions such as 'getting on my nerves', 'hitting a raw nerve' and 'having bad nerves' bear witness to this. However, nerves are not only involved in bad news but in all types of communication throughout the body. Furthermore, nerves project *to* and *from* the brain and spinal cord, rather than, as implied by common expressions, being located *in* the brain.

Nociceptively triggered pain has been closely researched over the years and the specific regions of the brain that are triggered into relatively high levels of activity by noxious stimuli have been identified and are termed the pain matrix. The nerves that convey nociceptive information to the spinal cord have been identified, as have the parts of the spinal cord engaged with this information.

3.6.3 The brain and types of trigger to pain

The kind of evidence presented so far leads to a representation of pain arising from the two types of trigger: nociceptive and psychogenic. Both of these excite the pain matrix, as shown in Figure 3.4. Activity within the pain matrix is felt as the conscious sensation of pain.

Figure 3.4a represents nociceptively triggered pain. The pain matrix is triggered by noxious stimuli (via what is termed the 'sensory route'). The inputs from

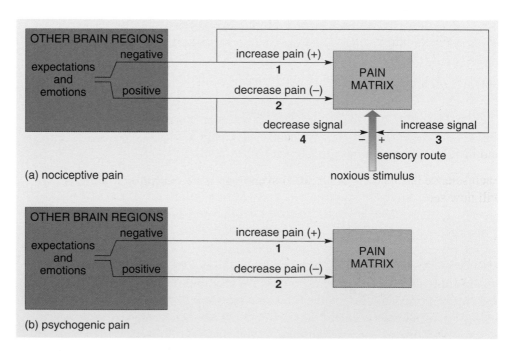

Figure 3.4 Triggers to pain. (a) Nociceptive and (b) psychogenic. Arrows 1 and 2 represent direct effects on the pain matrix, whereas arrows 3 and 4 represent influences on the sensory route, i.e. the flow of information from the noxious stimulus to the pain matrix.

'other brain regions', which act directly on the pain matrix, are represented by arrows 1 and 2. These inputs arise from such things as emotions, expectations and interpretations of pain. When they are negative, they can make pain more *intense* (indicated by the plus sign associated with arrow 1). Psychogenic factors such as stress and depression appear to act via this route. Conversely, positive emotions and psychological treatments can *lower* nociceptively triggered pain (indicated by the minus sign associated with arrow 2).

In addition to the direct effect on the pain matrix, the 'other brain regions' also affect the sensory route to the pain matrix, i.e. they affect information conveyed via nerves. This is indicated by arrow 3 (the plus sign indicates strengthening the sensory signal) and arrow 4 (the minus sign indicates weakening the sensory signal).

Figure 3.4b shows psychogenically triggered pain: complex emotional processing triggers the pain matrix in the absence of any nociceptive input. Social triggers such as disruption to a relationship act in this way. As a first approximation, the pain matrix is shown as the same in the two cases of (a) and (b). Of course, it might well not be identical but the evidence points to some overlap in the brain regions activated under the two conditions.

3.7 The study of mind and consciousness

3.7.1 General points

So far, to understand pain, we have described such things as the brain and nerves. We also noted that the conscious mind is involved with the experience of pain. So, how does the electrical activity of the brain give rise to the conscious mind? The truth is that absolutely no one knows! However, the book will proceed on the basis of the general assumption that the mind is the product of the activity of the brain.

Psychobiology attempts to link the operations of the mind to the physical basis of this processing in the brain. Some of this processing is carried out at an unconscious level, so, by definition, we do not have conscious insight into it. Other activities of the mind correspond to our conscious awareness. This section will look at the division between unconscious and conscious aspects of the mind and its relevance to understanding pain.

Each science has its own jargon and psychology is no exception to this, as you will now see.

3.7.2 Cognition

The term **cognition** refers to certain kinds of activity with which the brain is engaged, i.e. the processing of information that is summarised by the term 'mind'. Such processing is said to involve **cognitive processes**, e.g. thinking, memory and reasoning (as in interpreting the meaning of a pain). Psychologists can pose cognitive tasks to people, such as trying to count backwards in units of 7 from 879, and observe which parts of the brain are particularly active when they do this. Another cognitive task would be to imagine oneself on a tropical island and strolling along the beach there. By posing cognitive tasks, researchers build up a picture of how different aspects of mind relate to the underlying activity taking place in the brain.

Earlier, we mentioned distraction techniques for reducing pain, which are also termed 'cognitive interventions'. For example, therapists try to teach 'tricks' for diverting attention from chronic pain. Also, cognitive processes interpret the meaning of pain and some types of therapy target this meaning (described later). For example, patients have expectations about the efficacy of therapy. They try to reduce the impact of pain in various ways, such as giving themselves silent messages of the kind 'think positive – it will not last for ever' or 'just try to trust the doctors'.

3.7.3 Affect

The term **affect** is used (as a noun, pronounced *ah*-fect, with the stress on the first syllable) to refer to the dimension of positive and negative feelings. Recall that in Table 3.1 the term 'affective' was used to describe this dimension. In psychology, 'positive affect' corresponds to happiness and pleasure, whereas 'negative affect' corresponds to aversion, e.g. pain, depression and disgust. Between the extremes, there is a gradual change passing through 'zero affect', where the experience is neither pleasurable nor aversive.

3.7.4 Minds, consciousness and unconscious processing

This section considers the kind of cognition that is associated with conscious awareness and also that which is performed unconsciously. Now attempt Activity 3.2.

Activity 3.2   A thought experiment

Allow one or two minutes

At this point, please stop reading for a minute or two and describe the current contents of your conscious mind, that is to say, what is in your 'mind's eye' moment-by-moment?

You might have kept your thoughts unwavering with the science of pain. Perhaps more likely, your thoughts wandered – did I remember to invite the cat in for the night? I could just have one more cup of coffee…

Across a population of readers, Activity 3.2 will doubtless have generated a rich variety of idiosyncratic 'streams of consciousness'. However, what is probably common is that your conscious minds will be engaged with *one* different thing *after* another. It appears that different thoughts compete for access to consciousness. If you are unfortunate enough to be experiencing pain, then this might well be prioritised as the dominant content of consciousness. This means that other events (e.g. remembering to cancel the milk) will be placed at a disadvantage in terms of gaining access to your attention and conscious mind.

◆ Does such prioritisation of pain make any sense in terms of adaptive value?

◆ It would appear to do so in general. Pain is often 'telling you' that something requires urgent and dedicated attention. Seen in an evolutionary context, survival could depend upon taking the appropriate action.

◆ Look at Figure 3.5 and describe what you see.

◆ The chances are that you will see *either* a vase *or* two royal heads but not both of these simultaneously. Your conscious perception will alternate between the two possible interpretations.

This example illustrates two important things about consciousness. First, there is competition for conscious awareness, with one perception and then the other tending to grab control. Secondly, conscious processing tries to 'make sense'. There is either a vase or two heads, each of which is a rational interpretation of the world, but there is not a mixture of the two. Competition of information for entering consciousness is central to therapies for pain such as those that involve distraction of attention, as you will see in Chapter 7.

Now consider your experiences when observing the flow of your consciousness in Activity 3.2. Just as revealing as what entered your conscious mind, is what probably did *not* enter. Did you have thoughts about the pressure of the chair against your back or the floor under your feet or the pressure of a shoe? Why were such thoughts unlikely to enter consciousness? Information on these stimuli is available all the time to your brain, as you can instantly check now by focusing your conscious mind on it. Doubtless, you can now feel such things as the pressure of the chair or of a shoe. However, information on them is not normally prioritised since it is not important. It is processed at an *unconscious* level and, only if you deliberately focus on it, does it reach consciousness. By contrast, pain can command attention even against determined efforts to resist it.

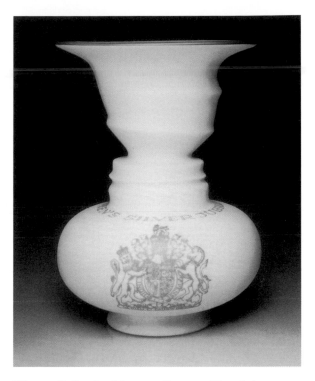

Figure 3.5   Ambiguous figure of heads/vase. (Source: Porzellan manufaktur Staffelstein)

So, conscious awareness represents a limited subset of all the information available to the brain. The rationale of psychological therapy for pain is to try to stop nociceptive information from dominating consciousness with the sensation of pain, even though such information is potentially able to do this.

When you observed the contents of conscious awareness, did information on internal events such as the movement of food along the gut enter awareness? It probably did not, unless there was some disturbance to such a process. Yet, the brain is involved with the control of digestion and other internal processes. Information on these processes is sent to the brain.

People have little or no conscious control over such internal processes. Perhaps it is just as well that they don't. So many people make such an awful mess of many of the activities over which they do have conscious control, e.g. by smoking and drinking too much and not getting enough sleep. Just imagine the chaos that would result if humans had full conscious control over the range of internal activities such as heart rate and stomach emptying!

The conclusion is that much information processing is carried out at a quite unconscious level, i.e. people have no conscious insight into it.

In order to understand brain, mind and behaviour, as exemplified by pain, you will first need to understand something of the structure and function of the body, and so Chapter 4 turns to this. Then, Chapter 5 looks in more detail at the brain, spinal cord and nerves, and how they all work.

Summary of Chapter 3

3.1 Viewed in terms of its evolutionary origins, nociceptive pain has adaptive value; it helps to protect the body from damage. However, not all instances of pain exhibited these days can necessarily be understood in terms of an adaptive function.

3.2 The study of pain involves trying to fit the subjective experience of the sufferer to objective measurements of the reactions of body and behaviour.

3.3 There is variation in pain sensitivity between individuals corresponding, to some extent, to psychological differences.

3.4 There are cultural differences in how pains are interpreted and expressed.

3.5 The brain is the basis of mental experience, including that of pain. The experience of pain corresponds to increased activity of the brain's 'pain matrix'. Information from other brain regions can modify this activity. Information from the body to the brain is conveyed through nerves and the spinal cord.

3.6 The conscious mind represents only part of the activity of the brain. There is some competition between events for access to conscious awareness.

Learning outcomes for Chapter 3

After studying this chapter and its associated activities, you should be able to:

LO 3.1 Define and use, or recognise definitions and applications of, each of the terms printed in **bold** in the text. (Questions 3.1, 3.2 and 3.3)

LO 3.2 Relate pain to the expressions 'adaptive value' and 'evolutionary trade-off'. (Question 3.1)

LO 3.3 Explain what is meant by claiming that pain usually has both subjective and objective aspects and give examples to illustrate this distinction. (Question 3.2 and DVD Activity 3.1)

LO 3.4 Present an argument that the brain forms the basis of mental experience. (Question 3.3)

LO 3.5 Explain why insight into consciousness is essential for understanding pain. (Question 3.3 and DVD Activity 3.1)

Self-assessment questions for Chapter 3

You also had the opportunity to demonstrate LOs 3.3 and 3.5 by answering questions in DVD Activity 3.1.

Question 3.1 (LOs 3.1 and 3.2)

Explain the adaptive value of (a) nociceptive pain and (b) psychogenic pain.

Question 3.2 (LOs 3.1 and 3.3)

Which of the following are (a) subjective measures, (b) objective measures or (c) proxy measures of pain? (Note: a measure can be both objective and proxy.)

(i) the number of painkillers prescribed over a 10-year period,

(ii) an abnormally high heart rate;

(iii) a score of 50 on a pain rating scale.

Question 3.3 (LOs 3.1, 3.4 and 3.5)

What evidence suggests that the brain forms the basis of the sensation of pain?

4   HOW THE BODY WORKS

As was described in the context of Figure 3.3, information on a disturbance to the body travels from the site of disturbance along nerves to the spinal cord and then to the brain. If the disturbance is sufficient, the brain triggers the sensation of pain and action is taken to oppose the disturbance.

Of course, the brain and nerves do not exist in isolation. They exist within a body that contains many other components such as the heart, stomach, liver and blood vessels. There is a complex interdependence between all of these parts. If things go wrong in one, there can be serious implications for all. The working of any part and the whole body depends upon the interactions between these parts. Thus, pain can be best understood in terms of its role in the overall organisation of the body, this being the theme of Chapter 4.

This chapter introduces some of the principal foundations of the branch of biology that is termed **physiology**: the study of the relationship between structure and function of body systems.

4.1   Body systems

There are various ways of describing the working of the body. For convenience of description and explanation of what different parts do, the body can be divided into **body systems**. A system is characterised by a combination of parts that serve a particular role. Some body systems will be familiar to you already. The circulatory system consists of the heart, blood and the veins and arteries that contain the blood, and it performs the role of circulating the blood around the body. The respiratory system consists of the lungs and air passages that lead to them, as well as the control exerted over breathing.

The principal concern here will be the **nervous system** (Figure 3.3). The nervous system is made up from the brain, the spinal cord and nerves located throughout the body.

The nervous system controls behaviour and mental life, as well as coordinating the body's physiology. For example, the nervous system is responsible for the detection of events in the world, such as lights and sounds, and the interpretation of them. When pain is felt, it is because of events happening within the brain. Of course, these brain events might be triggered initially by a rotting tooth or a thorn in the foot, and information on this is conveyed to the brain, but it is the brain that produces the feeling of pain. Acting via the spinal cord and nerves, the brain also exerts control over the muscles that move the body around, e.g. in response to pain. The nervous system is also responsible for actions such as regulating the body's temperature and the movement of food along the gut.

The value of looking at the nervous system in the context of the whole body is clear: the systems of the body are *tightly interdependent*. Life is only possible provided that a number of conditions in the body, such as its temperature, are kept relatively stable. Communication, coordination and integration between the parts of the body are vital and a primary role of the nervous system is to achieve this. For example, the brain needs to be informed of what is happening throughout the body and be able to influence events throughout all the other body systems.

The respiratory system is the topic of another book in this series *Chronic Obstructive Pulmonary Disease: A Forgotten Killer* (Midgley, 2008)

The body comprises a number of **organs**, such as the heart, lungs, kidneys and brain. An organ is a complex structure in the body serving a particular function. An organ is made up of billions of individual building blocks termed 'cells'. These are organised into different *tissues*, e.g. muscle tissue and nerve tissue. As an example, Figure 3.3 showed the nervous *system*, two *organs* (brain and spinal cord) and some *tissue* (e.g. that forming nerves).

For all body parts (including those of the nervous system) to function correctly, temperature, amongst many other features of the body, needs to be maintained within tight limits. In turn, maintenance of this temperature is critically dependent upon the activity of the nervous system. Similarly, the water and oxygen levels of the body need to be held within tight limits for the body to be able to function.

4.1.1 The fluid environment of the body

All the processes of life take place within the body's 'fluid environment'. Water permeates all the spaces of the body. Each part of the body, within cells and in spaces between them, is made up of this 'fluid environment'. The most obvious fluid part of the body is the water content of the blood, which gives the blood its liquidity, so it can flow through the blood vessels. But other regions of the body, such as the skin, also contain a large percentage of water.

The water of the body, whether that of the blood or skin or wherever, contains substances dissolved in it, such as nutrients and oxygen.

4.2 Cells

Cells are the basic structural units of all organisms. A given type of cell has some *specific* properties peculiar to where it is situated and the role that it serves there (Figure 4.1a). Though there are differences between types of cell, they all share certain *general* properties, no matter what form they take or where in the body they are located. For example, like all the other parts of the body, the cells of the nervous system are composed of about 60% water. Most types of cell contain a *nucleus*, where the genetic material is housed.

Figure 4.1b is a schematic representation of a few of the cells of the body. Each cell is to some extent a self-contained unit. It is surrounded by a 'cell membrane' that allows some substances to pass across easily and others only with difficulty or not at all. The composition of chemicals on the inside of the cell is somewhat different from that on the outside. Nutrients (e.g. glucose) and oxygen are brought to each cell in the blood, and waste products (e.g. carbon dioxide) are excreted from each cell (i.e. passed out across the cell membrane) and carried away in the blood or other fluids surrounding the cell.

The type of cell that will principally occupy us here is found in the nervous system and is given a special name: **neuron** (see Figure 4.1a). Billions of neurons are located in the brain and other regions of the nervous system and they come in a variety of different shapes and sizes. Note the part of the neuron termed the **axon**. Very many axons, together with other types of cell, form a nerve. Neurons are distinguished by the specialised role that they serve: to communicate and

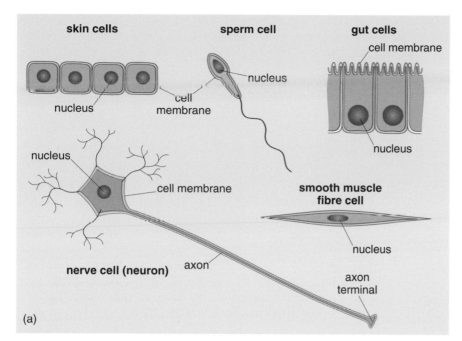

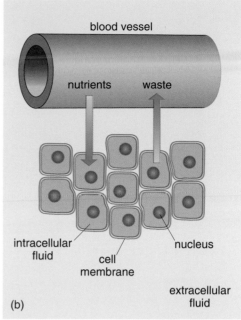

Figure 4.1 Cells. (a) Diagrammatic representation of some human cells of different kinds. (b) A simplified sketch of some cells of the body together with a nearby blood vessel. (Source: Eysenck, 1998, Figure 2.1, p. 25). Note: The diagram is not drawn to scale.

process information. To understand this, you will need to know a little more detail about how cells communicate as described in Box 4.1.

Box 4.1 (Explanation) Communication at the cell surface

Cell membranes act as 'switchboards' in a communication network of daunting complexity. Cells are constantly sending and receiving signals across the cell membrane, which either modify the activity inside the cell or change the conditions outside. The transmission of information on tissue damage in the body and the experience of pain depend upon such signalling.

Cells can secrete a variety of different signalling chemicals into the fluid outside the cell and these convey their chemical message to other cells. How is a chemical able to signal to the correct cells and to no others? The answer lies in what is termed a **lock-and-key interaction** (Figure 4.2, overleaf).

The chemical compounds that we describe here are made up of very many small units termed 'molecules'. The meaning of this term will be described in a moment but for now just consider that it refers to a very small unit into which these chemicals can be divided. In Figure 4.2, note the signalling molecule and the receptor embedded in the cell membrane.

Each signalling molecule has a highly specific three-dimensional shape. In addition, the surface of the signalling molecule not only has this three-dimensional shape in physical space, it also has a characteristic distribution of *electrons* – the smallest atomic particles, which carry a negative electrical charge.

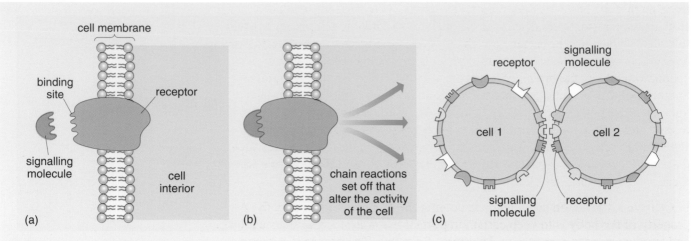

Figure 4.2 (a) and (b) Diagrammatic representation of stages in a 'lock-and-key' interaction between a 'free-floating' signalling molecule and the binding site of a receptor that is embedded in a cell membrane. (c) Cells in close contact can send and receive signals simultaneously when signalling molecules in the membrane of each cell bind to receptors on the other cell. There are commonly many different signalling molecules and receptors on the same cell, either on its surface or in its internal structure.

This part of the signalling molecule (Figure 4.2a) is analogous to a 'key'. The shape and electron distribution on the surface of the signalling molecule exactly fit a 'complementary image' of itself known as the *binding site* on the surface of a **receptor**, as in Figure 4.2b. This is like the lock. The two surfaces fit together so precisely that — like a key in a lock — no other combination of molecules will result in the transmission of the correct signal.

Many of the molecules that project from the outer membrane of every cell are actually receptors. When a receptor encounters a signalling molecule to which it can bind (that is, form a very close, though transient contact), the binding event sets off a chain reaction which leads ultimately to a change in the activity of the cell that received the signal (Figure 4.2b). In the example in Figure 4.2a and b, the receptor is part of the structure of a membrane and the signalling molecule is 'free-floating' in the fluid outside the cell. However, both receptor and signalling molecule can be embedded in a cell membrane and this provides a mechanism to transmit messages back and forth between adjacent cells — a process called 'cell-to-cell communication' (as in Figure 4.2c).

4.3 Homeostasis

Life is full of examples of both change and stability. Consider your growth from a newborn and the emergence of sexual maturity. This represents enormous changes in the structure of the body and the kind of information processing done by the brain. The female menstrual cycle exemplifies another form of change over time. Yet any such changes are only possible against a background of stability. For example, with luck, your body temperature has probably only deviated very slightly from a value of 37 °C. This is even in the face of extreme external temperatures, which have the potential to either lower body temperature or send it soaring. Similarly, the water content of your body has probably not strayed too far from its normal value. How is such constancy possible?

Imagine that the body temperature of a human starts to rise as a result of strenuous exercise. Specialised neurons that are sensitive to temperature detect this rise. They signal information to the brain and the brain triggers the automatic reaction of secreting sweat onto the skin. This serves to cool the body by evaporation. Also, the brain generates the sensation of thirst and the tendency to take cool drinks and move into the shade (unless the vanity of a sun-tan dominates the person's priorities). Conversely, imagine that a person is exposed to cold and body temperature falls. Specialised neurons detect the fall and shivering is automatically triggered, which means a vibration of muscles such that heat is generated. Also, if possible, the person will tend to move to a warmer location and put on extra clothes.

In each case, the action taken tends to counter the disturbance to the body. A property of the body is to keep certain important features at a near constant level and to take action in response to departures from this. The property is known as **homeostasis** and is maintained by a process termed **negative feedback**. Why the term *feedback*? Figure 4.3 illustrates the general principle by means of the example of temperature regulation. The brain's action is based upon a comparison of the actual body temperature against an 'optimal value', which is set by the brain. When body temperature deviates from the set level, the brain issues commands, such as to sweat or shiver, according to whether the body is too hot or too cold. These actions then change body temperature. Information on body temperature (in various parts of the body) is *fed* back to the brain. Why the term *negative* feedback? Any deviation from normal tends to trigger a counter-reaction that opposes the deviation. The deviation tends to be self-negating ('self-correcting'), hence the term 'negative' and the minus sign in Figure 4.3. The minus sign refers to the process of reducing the deviation until the optimal level is restored.

In a sense, pain also exemplifies the principle of homeostasis and negative feedback.

◆ In what way?

◆ Maintaining the body intact and stable in the face of threats, such as infectious agents and tissue damage, is vital to survival. Pain indicates that something is wrong. It triggers action of a kind that tends to correct (i.e. 'negate') the disturbance.

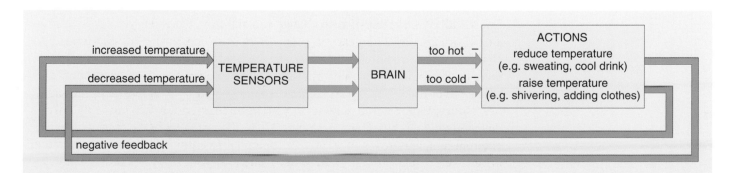

Figure 4.3 The principle of negative feedback, as applied to temperature regulation.

In maintaining the homeostasis of the body, the endocrine system has a vital role to play, described next.

4.4 The endocrine system

In addition to the nervous system, another means of communication within the body is by the **endocrine system** and it involves chemical signalling molecules termed **hormones**. They exemplify signalling of the kind shown in Figure 4.2a and b. Hormones are made by specialised cells in what are termed 'endocrine glands' at various locations in the body (Figure 4.4). A hormone is a chemical that is secreted by an endocrine gland into the blood at one site. At another site (the target), the hormone exerts an effect on cells that have specialised receptors for it. These receptors have a shape and surface electron distribution that is complementary to that of the hormone, so they fit together like a lock and key.

See Figure 4.5a. Imagine that it shows the hormone, epinephrine, and one of its targets in the body: the heart. Note the shape that is used to represent the molecules of this hormone (a filled triangle; in reality the shape is much more complex) and the correspondence with the shape of the receptors. In response to threats, e.g. social challenge or noxious stimuli, epinephrine is released in large

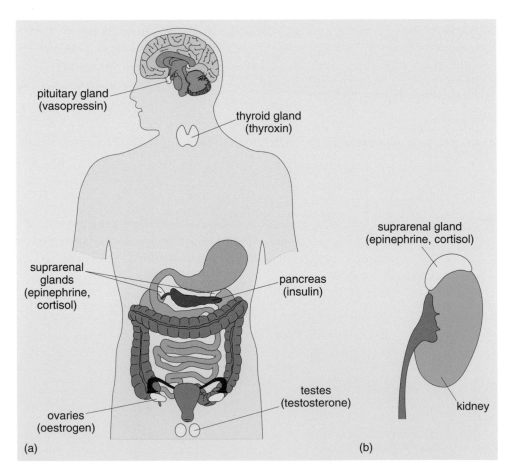

(a)   (b)

Figure 4.4   The location of the major endocrine glands and some of the hormones they produce.

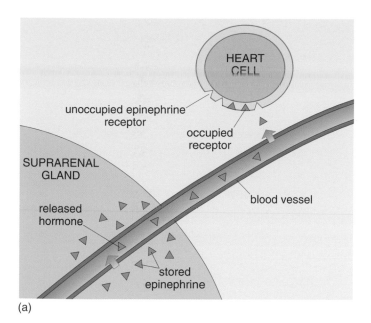

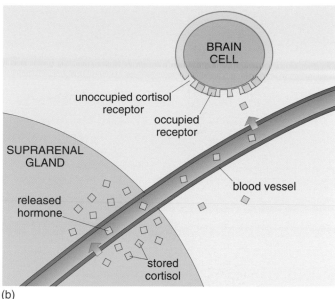

Figure 4.5 Schematic representation of two hormones and their targets: (a) epinephrine and its receptors on cells in the heart; (b) cortisol and its receptors on cells in the brain.

amounts from the inner region of the suprarenal gland (formerly known as the 'adrenal gland') into the bloodstream. It is sometimes described as the 'flight, fright or fight hormone'.

Epinephrine travels around the body until it occupies receptors on the cells of the muscles of the heart, amongst many other places. By means of the hormone's action when it binds to its receptors, the hormone contributes to the acceleration in heart rate at such times.

Figure 4.5b shows the action of another hormone: cortisol. It is released from the outer layer of the suprarenal gland in response to such things as stress, physical trauma and social loss. Its target is, amongst other sites in the body, neurons of the brain involved with processing emotional information. Note the different shape used to represent this hormone as compared with epinephrine. Again, there is a lock-and-key relationship between the chemical and its receptors. This gives *specificity*, i.e. only this hormone can bind to its specific receptor and trigger the resulting activity in the target cell (see also Box 4.1).

Amongst other things, hormones help to preserve homeostasis. For example, when the level of body water falls, a hormone termed vasopressin, is released from the pituitary gland (see Figure 4.4). It occupies receptors on the kidney cells and thereby generates signals that slow up the production of urine, so that the body retains more water.

◆ Which feedback principle does this example illustrate?

◆ Negative feedback. Vasopressin 'negates' the potential threat of a low level of fluids in the body.

So much for some general principles of physiology, in the next chapter we will apply some of these to understanding the nervous system.

Summary of Chapter 4

4.1   As a convenience for description and explanation, the body can be divided into *systems* such as the endocrine system and the nervous system. Each body system consists of *organs* composed of *tissues*, made up of many types of *cell*.

4.2   The cells of the body are each surrounded by a cell membrane. The membrane contains receptors which can be occupied by signalling molecules.

4.3   A major type of cell found in the nervous system is the neuron.

4.4   The tendency of the body to maintain such states as its temperature within tight limits is termed 'homeostasis'. Deviation from the normal value triggers corrective action, termed negative feedback.

4.5   The endocrine system employs hormones for communication and receptors to which the hormone binds like a key in a lock.

Learning outcomes for Chapter 4

After studying this chapter and its associated activities, you should be able to:

LO 4.1   Define and use, or recognise definitions and applications of, each of the terms printed in **bold** in the text. (Questions 4.1, 4.2 and 4.3)

LO 4.2   Describe links between the nervous system, negative feedback and homeostasis. (Question 4.1)

LO 4.3   Explain how pain illustrates the principle of homeostasis. (Question 4.2)

LO 4.4   By means of one or two specific examples, describe what is meant by a hormone and a lock-and-key interaction. (Question 4.3)

Self-assessment questions for Chapter 4

Question 4.1 (LOs 4.1 and 4.2)

How does drinking in response to dehydration illustrate the principles of homeostasis and negative feedback?

Question 4.2 (LOs 4.1 and 4.3)

The maintenance of stability of body temperature and the reaction to pain are rather different properties. However, in terms of homeostasis and negative feedback, identify an important feature that they share.

Question 4.3 (LOs 4.1 and 4.4)

(a) How can the terms 'lock' and 'key' be applied to epinephrine? (b) How does the action of epinephrine aid survival?

5   THE NERVOUS SYSTEM

This chapter looks at one particular system of the body, the nervous system, since it is fundamental to trying to explain pain. To understand the nervous system, we will call on some general principles of physiology (Chapter 4), as well as introduce some physiological principles that apply specifically to the nervous system.

Figure 5.1a should remind you of the structure of the nervous system. As part of the nervous system, the brain and spinal cord together are termed the **central nervous system,** abbreviated as the **CNS**. All the nervous system that is not located in the CNS forms the **peripheral nervous system**.

It is now necessary to take apart a nerve (only metaphorically speaking!) to see how it serves its function in the transmission of information.

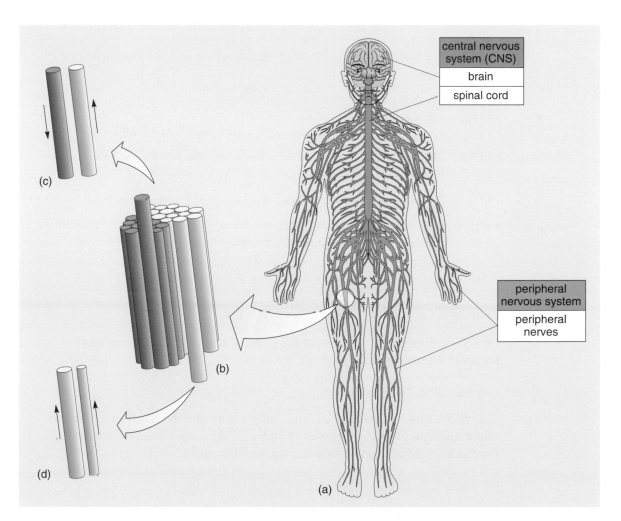

Figure 5.1   The nervous system. (a) Overall system; (b) a segment cut from a nerve; (c) identification of the role of axons; (d) further classification of the role of some axons.

5.1 Nerves, neurons and axons

Figure 5.1a indicates a short segment being cut from a nerve; this segment is shown in Figure 5.1b. A nerve looks something like a bundle of wires that form a cable. These wire-like structures are the axons and each one forms part of a neuron. Each axon is specialised to carry a particular kind of information. In Figure 5.1b, simply for the convenience of explanation, some axons are indicated by the colour light green and some by the colour dark green. Suppose, as indicated in Figure 5.1c, that all of those axons coloured light green convey information from the outer areas of the body to the spinal cord. By contrast, imagine that all those coloured dark green convey information in the opposite direction, i.e. to the periphery.

◆ What type of information is carried in the light green axons?

◆ Information on tissue damage ('nociceptive information'), temperature and harmless touch.

◆ Suppose that the axons coloured dark green convey information to muscles. What does this information signal?

◆ It carries commands from the spinal cord on the amount that the muscle needs to contract.

Now looking more closely at the axons coloured light green in Figure 5.1d, you can see that there are two types of axon that convey information from the outer areas of the body to the spinal cord. The thin axons convey information on tissue damage whereas the thicker ones convey information on such qualities as warmth, cold and light touch.

5.2 Types of neuron

Figure 5.2a and b shows two types of whole neuron, represented both in grossly simplified form (left) and semi-realistically (right). The simplified representation is used later, in order to keep diagrams that involve several neurons manageable. Figure 5.2a shows a **sensory neuron**, one that responds to events in the world such as heat or tissue damage. The sensory ending detects such events. The single type of neuron shown in Figure 5.2b represents neurons that serve two roles, 'interneurons' and 'motor neurons', described in a moment. Figure 5.2c is a photograph of a single neuron within the brain.

To exemplify how different types of neurons can be found in combinations, see Figure 5.3. The axon of neuron 1, a sensory neuron, carries nociceptive information (i.e. information triggered by a noxious, potentially damaging stimulus) from the periphery (e.g. the foot) to the spinal cord (Figure 5.3b). Hence, in this special case, the sensory ending is termed a 'nociceptive ending'.

Figure 5.3b shows three different classes of neuron. Neurons serve various roles and can be classified according to this role. Those that convey information *from* the body outside the CNS *to* the CNS are the sensory neurons.

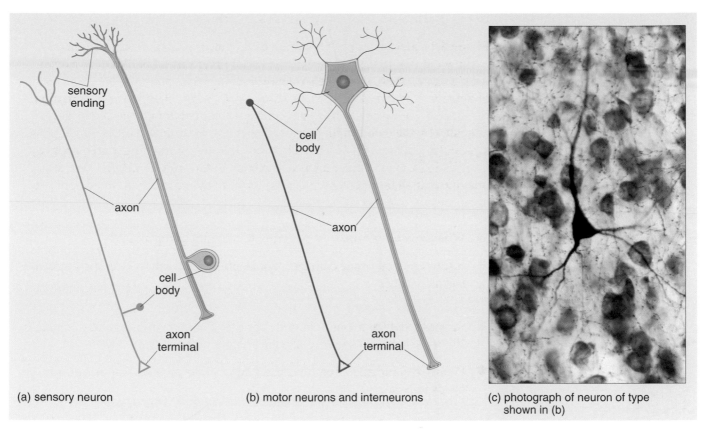

(a) sensory neuron

(b) motor neurons and interneurons

(c) photograph of neuron of type shown in (b)

Figure 5.2 (a) and (b) Representations of (a) a sensory neuron and (b) motor neurons and interneurons. Left: grossly simplified; right: semi-realistic. (c) Photograph of a single neuron (coloured black) within the brain. The cell bodies of other neurons can be seen as purple structures in the background. The neurons have been magnified approximately 350 times. (Photo: Paul Gabbott)

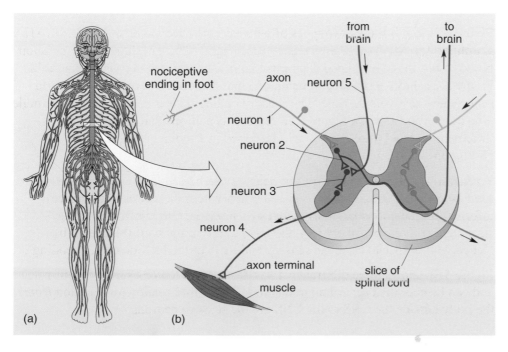

Figure 5.3 (a) The nervous system and (b) an enlarged slice through the spinal cord and some of the neurons found there.

◆ In Figure 5.3b, which of the numbered neurons is of this kind?

◆ Neuron 1.

Neurons that convey information *from* the CNS *to* the muscles are termed **motor neurons** and one is shown numbered in Figure 5.3b.

◆ Which neuron is this?

◆ Neuron 4.

Neuron 4 takes the form shown in Figure 5.2b. When motor neurons are activated, muscles are caused to exert force. In the case of neurons 1 and 4, note the single long structure: the axon.

All of the neurons of the body that are *neither* sensory neurons *nor* motor neurons are classified as **interneurons**. This is the most numerous type of neuron in the nervous system and consists of many billions deep in the brain and spinal cord. It also takes the form shown in Figure 5.2b.

◆ In Figure 5.3b, which of the numbered neurons are interneurons?

◆ Neurons 2, 3 and 5.

Note that neurons *almost* touch each other but not quite, e.g. neuron 1 almost touches neuron 2 (we will return to this 'gap' between neurons later). Neuron 2 is within the spinal cord and it has an axon that branches, with one branch extending to the brain. It is by means of neurons such as this one that nociceptive information indicating tissue damage reaches the brain.

5.3   The role of neurons

This section describes some of the roles of neurons in communication and processing of information about tissue damage and other important information in the body.

5.3.1 The role of neurons in reflexes

Have you ever put your hand or foot into very hot water or onto a sharp object and instantly pulled it back, crying out in pain? You might have imagined that the heat or sharp object triggered the pain, which then caused you to move your hand away. Of course, the damaging stimulus triggers pain but this pain cannot explain the instant reaction, which is termed a **reflex**. Rather, the reflex is triggered automatically by the stimulus and is well under way even before you have the conscious sensation of pain. It is said to be triggered 'unconsciously'.

Figure 5.3b showed a series of neurons, which link the surface of the foot to the muscles involved in pulling the foot from the noxious stimulus, i.e. forming the reflex. The sequence of neurons 1 → 2 → 3 → 4 → muscle forms a relay and is the neural basis of this reflex. Note that the brain does not form a part of this particular reflex.

The term 'neural' is an adjective that means anything to do with neurons.

A 'nociceptive neuron', represented here as 'neuron 1', detects tissue damage at its nociceptive ending at the foot. The neuron is said to be *excited* when damage happens at the nociceptive ending (or an impact is near to causing damage). In reality, being bound together, axons of many such neurons project from a given region of the periphery (e.g. the foot) to the spinal cord.

The term 'reflex' is used to cover automatic reactions that occur in response to particular trigger stimuli. Another example of a reflex is the contraction of the pupils of the eyes when someone shines a bright light into your face. (The brain is part of this particular reflex).

5.3.2 The role in pain

Suppose that someone treads heavily on your foot. A brief moment later you feel pain and say 'ouch'! The initial trigger to the sequence of events was at the foot but a message has quickly got to the brain and the pain sensation is triggered there. Your brain then communicates to your vocal apparatus and you make the exclamation. So, how is a message sent from the foot up to the brain?

Consider a sequence of neurons shown in Figure 5.3b and which is involved in pain. Excitation triggered by the noxious stimulus is conveyed along the length of the axon of neuron 1 and then it is passed on to neuron 2. This much is common with the reflex just described. But notice that a branch of neuron 2 conveys the message up to the brain.

In reality, many axons in parallel carry nociceptive information along the spinal cord, and thereby up to the brain. Within the spinal cord a different term from 'nerve' is used to describe a bundle of axons: a tract. In the brain, collections of millions of neurons generate the experience of pain, which then links to the vocal reaction. How neurons convey information will be explained in a moment. Box 5.1 gives an example of what can happen when they malfunction.

> **Box 5.1** (Enrichment) The relevance of nociceptive neurons to leprosy
>
> Chapter 3 described the adaptive value of taking action in response to tissue damage or the threat of it. Understanding the normal role of nociceptive neurons can help to illuminate an important feature of the disease of leprosy (also known as Hansen's disease).
>
> Leprosy is caused by the invasion of the body by a microbe (*Mycobacterium leprae*). This tends to cause particular damage to peripheral regions of the nervous system, including nociceptive neurons. As a result of the loss of nociception, protective action is no longer taken in response to the minor cuts and abrasions to hands and feet that are a feature of everyday life. In other words, the person loses the warning signal of pain. Hence, this damage tends to get worse, with ulceration and a loss of tissue.
>
> These days leprosy exists mainly in Asia, Brazil and Africa, and is associated with poor hygiene and sanitation. In earlier centuries, it was widespread in Europe.

So, our defence against noxious stimuli is made up of two different systems that act in a coordinated way:

1   Reflexes, which act rapidly, unconsciously and automatically.

2   The control exerted on the basis of pain. Pain allows for slower and more flexible ('consciously thought-through') reactions to noxious stimuli.

Neurons are involved in all forms of communication in the body, not just those involved with detecting tissue damage and triggering pain and defensive reflexes.

5.4   How do neurons perform their role?

You have now seen some examples of neurons and the role that they serve. We spoke of 'neurons being excited' and 'information conveyed in neurons'. How do neurons perform this role by means of 'being excited'? How is information conveyed in neurons? The key to understanding this is to examine the electrical properties of some of the chemical components of the body and how these properties are exploited by cells for communication. First, you need to understand some basic terms and concepts.

5.4.1 Elements, atoms, molecules and ions

All matter, whether it is in a living organism, such as a tree or a person, or in non-living material, such as the rocks and the atmosphere, is composed of chemical **elements** – a substance that is composed of just one type of atom.

There are about 90 different elements in nature and among the most familiar are the most abundant constituents of living things: oxygen, carbon, nitrogen and hydrogen, which together form over 90 per cent of the mass of every organism. Each element is built up from very small particles known as **atoms**. Elements and atoms are not changed by *chemical* reactions, they remain intact.

Atoms are composed of many fundamental particles. Within an atom there are equal numbers of positively charged and negatively charged particles. The negatively charged particles are called **electrons** and the positively charged particles are called **protons**. The charges on a proton and on an electron are equal and opposite. Because the numbers of protons and electrons in an atom are the same, an atom is electrically neutral, that is, it has no net electrical charge. The third type of particle is the neutron which has the same mass as a proton but which carries no charge. One element is distinguished from another only by the number of protons (and thus electrons) that each atom contains. For example, hydrogen, the simplest atom contains one proton and one electron only. In contrast, sodium possesses eleven protons and eleven electrons (and twelve neutrons).

A proton is approximately 2000 times as heavy as an electron. The electrons are to be found moving around the outside of the dense core of the atom, the atomic nucleus, which contains the protons and neutrons.

Atoms tend to join together; an assembly of two or more types of atom in fixed proportions is known as a **chemical compound**. Some compounds are composed of **molecules** – two or more atoms held together by chemical bonds. The atoms in each molecule have a particular geometrical arrangement in relation to

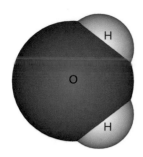

Figure 5.4 Model of a molecule of water consisting of one oxygen atom (O) joined to two hydrogen atoms (H). In molecular models such as these, it is the convention to use standard colours to symbolise atoms of different elements: hydrogen is white and oxygen is red, as here.

each other, giving the molecule a characteristic three-dimensional shape. Molecules mostly contain atoms of more than one element, so, for example, water molecules are formed from two atoms of hydrogen and one atom of oxygen, written in the familiar chemical notation of H_2O (a representation of a water molecule is shown in Figure 5.4). Water is a very small molecule because it has only three atoms, but molecules can be millions of times larger than those of water and contain the atoms of several different elements. Some of the largest of these 'macromolecules' – the class termed *proteins* – are an essential part of the body.

The details of atomic structure need not concern you here, except in one respect, which is key to the transmission of electrical signals in neurons. The outer part of each atom is formed by the negatively charged electrons circulating around the positively charged central atomic nucleus. Under certain circumstances, an atom can gain an *extra* electron. In so doing, it will become negatively charged, because it has more negative charge in its outer layer than is counterbalanced by the positive charge in its nucleus.

◆ What will happen if an atom *loses* an electron?

◆ It will become *positively charged* because it has lost a negatively charged electron; the positive charge in the atom's nucleus now exceeds the negative charges of the surrounding electrons.

The general name for atoms that have become positively or negatively charged is **ion** (eye-on). For example, consider two ions that are essential for the functioning of the body, the sodium ion, written as Na^+ in chemical notation (sodium-plus *or* en-aye-plus) and the chloride ion (Cl^-, see-el-minus). In common table salt (sodium chloride, NaCl), the sodium and chloride ions are held together by the attraction of their opposite charges. On dissolving in water the constituent Na^+ and Cl^- ions of NaCl are separated because each ion is surrounded by water molecules. The movement of such electrically charged ions in the body make them very important in many biological processes.

The process of NaCl dissolving in water is described in more detail in another book in this series (Halliday and Davey, 2007).

You saw earlier that cells can secrete a variety of different signalling molecules, such as hormones, into the fluid outside the cell and these transmit their chemical message to other cells using a 'lock-and-key' interaction.

Each signalling molecule has a highly specific three-dimensional shape, resulting from the arrangement of the atoms from which it is formed. The atoms that form the surface of the signalling molecule, although they are not ions, do each carry a slightly different amount of electrical charge, some having slight positive charge, others are biased towards being negatively charged, and some are neutral. This means that the surface of the signalling molecule not only has a three-dimensional shape in physical space, it also has a characteristic charge profile – a unique pattern of electrical charges and neutral areas are distributed across its surface. The shapes and charges of the atoms on its surface exactly fit the binding site on the surface of the receptor molecule. The positive charges on one molecule are matched by negative charges on the other, and so on.

So, what have ions to do with how electrical signals arise and are transmitted? Recall the account given earlier of the cell membrane (Section 4.2). The fluid on each side contains ions. This membrane separates two rather different chemical environments on either side of the membrane. The fluid inside all the cells of the body is termed 'intracellular fluid' and that outside the cells is termed 'extracellular fluid'. The difference in the distribution of ions on either side of the membrane gives rise to a small **potential difference** (also known as a voltage) across the membrane of the cell. For a familiar example of a voltage, see Box 5.2.

Box 5.2 (Explanation) Electricity

In a household battery, a potential difference (or voltage) is generated by chemical means between the two terminals (Figure 5.5). If you were to take a voltmeter (an instrument that measures potential differences) and connect it to the terminals, it would register a voltage of, for example, 1.5 volts (Figure 5.5a) between the two terminals, one of which is marked positive (+) and the other negative (−). If you connect a light bulb via wires to the two terminals, charge will flow between them and the bulb will light up. The reason for this is that an electric current flows through the wire and the light bulb (Figure 5.5b).

In this case the current in the wire is carried by electrons travelling from the

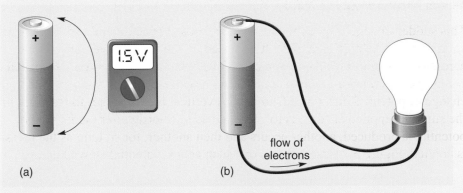

flow of electrons

(a)   (b)

Figure 5.5 Battery: (a) with voltage measuring apparatus and (b) connected to a light bulb.

negative terminal of the battery to the positive terminal, but in general terms current can be carried by any charged particle that can flow; in cells it is carried by the movement of ions.

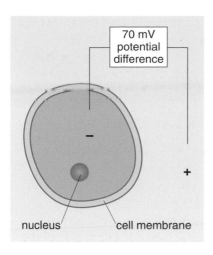

Figure 5.6 Diagram showing the potential difference (voltage) between the inside and outside of a living cell.

70 mV potential difference

nucleus   cell membrane

A potential difference is present across the cell membranes in the body (Figure 5.6). Some cells in non-human species (e.g. squid) are relatively enormous, which facilitates measurement of the potential difference. If you were to take a sensitive voltmeter and locate its very fine terminals, one on the inside and one on the outside of any cell, you would find a small potential difference. It is about 70 mV (millivolts), which means 70 thousandths of one volt. It is very small indeed compared with most of the voltage that we come across in everyday life, but it is the secret to the activity of the nervous system.

Changes in this voltage across the cell membrane are the signals that the nervous system uses to convey information within neurons. How is this done? Consider again someone treading hard on your toe and think of the neurons with the nociceptive endings of their axons in the toe. When the pressure is applied, there is a sudden change in the potential difference at the nociceptive ending, as in neuron 1 represented in Figure 5.3b.

This sudden change of potential difference across the cell membrane is termed an **action potential** (Figure 5.7). It is caused by the rapid movement of ions across 'ion channels' in the membrane of the cell. Note the neuron's so-called *resting potential* prior to the external stimulus (impact on the foot) and the rapid change of potential difference (shown as a vertical line or spike) in response to the stimulus applied at 'time zero', labelled as t_0. Shortly after the first action potential is produced, another occurs and then another, for so long as the pressure is applied. Figure 5.7 (inset) shows one such action potential slowed up in

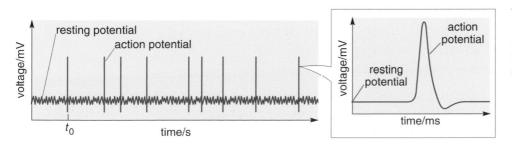

resting potential

action potential

voltage/mV

t_0 time/s

action potential

resting potential

voltage/mV

time/ms

Note that the horizontal scale in the inset to Figure 5.7 has changed to milliseconds (ms) to enable you to see the form of the action potential.

Figure 5.7 Record of activity in a neuron showing periods of resting and a number of action potentials, with one enlarged (inset).

Figure 5.8 Movement of an action potential along an axon. Events at different time points are described in the text.

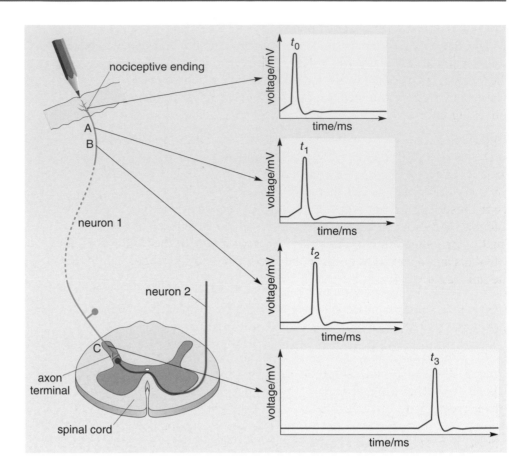

time, so you can see the shape of the change in potential difference with time. An action potential triggered at the nociceptive ending of the axon of a neuron travels the length of the axon all the way to the spinal cord.

Imagine how a neuron might be activated. In Figure 5.8, the axon of a neuron is activated by a sharp object pricking the skin at time zero (t_0), i.e. an action potential is generated at the nociceptive ending, and then travels along the axon of neuron 1. A fraction of a second later (time t_1) it has reached point A on the axon and then, a bit later still (time t_2), it reaches location B. By time t_3, the action potential has almost reached the axon terminal (C).

Events at the axon terminal, described in a moment, then trigger a change in the potential difference across the membrane of the next neuron (neuron 2). This next neuron in the sequence becomes 'excited' and another action potential arises there, and so on until the signal goes deep into the brain.

5.4.2 The language of the nervous system

The scientific convention is to write 'per second' as s^{-1}, which is pronounced as 's to the minus one'.

To illustrate the range of different sensory neurons, imagine that Figure 5.9a represents a neuron that is not particularly sensitive to tissue damage but is sensitive to warmth at its sensory ending. The sensory ending is located at a finger tip. Suppose that you put your finger in water at body temperature. Since the neuron is sensitive to warmth *above* body temperature, it will not be triggered into activity. So, the graph of action potentials shows no activity of any kind (Figure 5.9b).

Now you put the finger in water above body temperature (Figure 5.9c). This changes the electrical activity at the sensory ending and it produces an action potential (indicated by a vertical trace), which travels along the axon's length. The finger remains in the water and note that one action potential is shortly followed by another and then another. Each of them travels along the axon, conveying information to the brain concerning temperature at the finger.

Suppose that, during a one second period of observation, 5 such action potentials occur (Figure 5.9c). In other words the *frequency* (or, if you prefer the term, 'rate') of action potentials is 5 per second, abbreviated as 5 s^{-1}. Now you put your finger in water that is still warmer and observe what happens. You see the result shown in Figure 5.9d. In the one second period, now 10 action potentials are shown to occur. In other words, the frequency is now 10 s^{-1}. Finally, the temperature of the water is increased still further and more action potentials are observed to occur in the one-second period (Figure 5.9e). Now attempt Activity 5.1.

Activity 5.1   Constructing a graph

Allow about 15 minutes

Figure 5.10 is a blank sheet of graph paper with the axes already drawn and Table 5.1 (overleaf) gives some data points for plotting a graph of the relationship between temperature and the frequency of action potentials in a warm-sensitive neuron. At body temperature (37 °C) the frequency of action potentials is zero. You can now draw a graph relating temperature (along the horizontal axis) to the frequency of generation of action potentials (along the vertical axis) on Figure 5.10. Suppose that, at 40 °C, the frequency was 5 s^{-1} (Table 5.1). So, a line is projected upwards from this value on the horizontal axis and across to the value of 5 s^{-1} on the vertical axis. Similarly, at 45 °C, a line is projected upwards and across to 8 s^{-1}, and so on. When you have plotted all the data points, you can compare your graph with that shown in Figure 5.21, which appears at the end of the book.

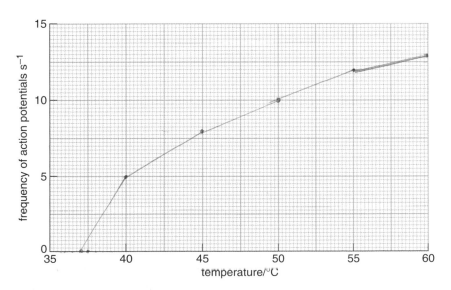

Figure 5.10   Graph for plotting data on activity of a warm-sensitive neuron at various temperatures.

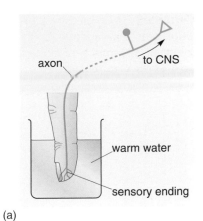

(a)

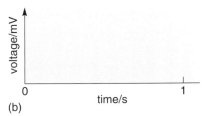

(b)

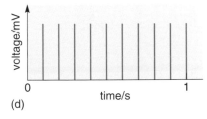

(c)

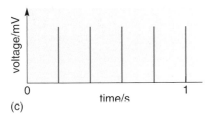

(d)

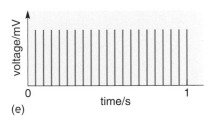

(e)

Figure 5.9   Activity in a warm-sensitive neuron. (a) Finger in water; (b) no reaction at body temperature; (c)–(e) the reaction to increasing temperatures is an increase in the frequency of action potentials.

Table 5.1 Data for plotting graph in Figure 5.10

Temperature/°C	Frequency of action potentials s^{-1}
37	0
40	5
45	8
50	10
55	12
60	13

As you can see, as temperature increases the neuron becomes increasingly 'excited'.

This example demonstrates the language of the nervous system: it *signals* temperature in terms of the frequency of action potentials. Your brain is able to *interpret* the increasing frequency of action potentials originating in warm-sensitive neurons as increasing degrees of warmth at the finger tip.

The class of neuron of primary interest to the discussion of pain is the nociceptive neuron. Increased frequency here would typically be interpreted as increased pain. Other neurons convey information to muscles.

◆ What is this class of neuron called?

◆ Motor neurons (Section 5.2).

Try clenching your fist but not too hard. The muscles controlling your fingers are activated by action potentials arising in the brain and conveyed out to the muscles. Now try clenching harder. This involves increased exertion of force by the muscles.

◆ How do you suppose that this is achieved?

◆ By an increase in the *frequency* of action potentials in the motor neurons that control the muscles (*Comment*: In Figure 5.3b, neuron 5 would convey such a command from the brain and thereby activate the motor neuron.)

Look back at Figure 5.3. With reference to neurons 1 and 2 in Figure 5.3b, the junction where neuron 1 communicates with neuron 2 is of crucial importance in the study of pain. This is because the capacity of neuron 1 to influence neuron 2 can vary. Several factors that are important to the study of pain influence this capacity. As one aspect, the junction can form a target for drugs that lower pain by reducing the chances that activity in neuron 1 can excite neuron 2. So, the next step is to look at the general properties of such junctions as they relate to neurons throughout the nervous system.

5.5 Synapses

5.5.1 The nature of synapses

As with the other adjacent cells shown in Figure 5.3b, neurons 1 and 2 *almost* make direct contact but not quite. However, across the minute gap between them, one neuron can influence another, e.g. neuron 1 influences neuron 2. How?

The junction where one neuron influences another cell is known as a **synapse** and one neuron is said to form a 'synaptic' link with another (Figure 5.11). You might like to imagine this as representing the junction of neurons 1 and 2 in Figure 5.3b. Note the small gap between neurons. With reference to this synapse, neuron 1, being before the gap, is defined as *presynaptic*. Neuron 2, being after the gap, is defined as *postsynaptic*. In Figure 5.11, note the chemical called a **neurotransmitter** that is stored at the axon terminal of the presynaptic neuron.

When an action potential reaches the axon terminal of the first neuron, it causes the release of neurotransmitter. This neurotransmitter crosses the gap very quickly and attaches to receptors on the membrane of the postsynaptic neuron. Note the shape of the molecules of neurotransmitter and the corresponding shape of the receptor, which have been drawn as interlocking partners. The neurotransmitter fits like a key in a lock.

◆ You have already met the lock-and-key analogy. To what did it refer?

◆ The general principle of communication at the cell surface (Box 4.1). As an example of this, the action of hormones and their receptors was described, e.g. epinephrine acting on cells in the heart muscle (Section 4.4).

When neurotransmitter molecules attach to their corresponding receptors, there is a change in the electrical activity of the second cell. In the specific case under

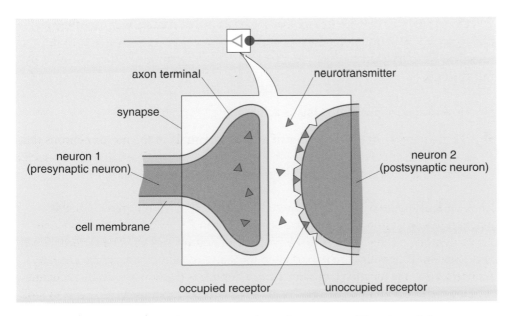

Figure 5.11 Diagrammatic representation of a synapse. The size of the neurotransmitter molecules and their receptors has been grossly exaggerated.

discussion, action potentials *tend to* be created in the second neuron as a result of the occupation of its receptors with neurotransmitter. These action potentials then carry the message further, e.g. in the case of Figure 5.3 towards the muscle and up to the brain. The caution 'tend to' will be explained later.

After attaching to the receptors on the postsynaptic neuron, the neurotransmitter is *inactivated* in one of two ways. This is shown in Figure 5.12. In some cases, the neurotransmitter is literally broken down. In other cases, it is taken back into the presynaptic neuron (from which it was released) and recycled. Thereby, the postsynaptic neuron is ready for the next signal.

◆ What would happen if the neurotransmitter were not removed from the synapse?

◆ It would activate the second neuron indefinitely regardless of the activity within the first neuron.

◆ So, information is transmitted *within* neurons by which means?

◆ Electrical, i.e. action potentials.

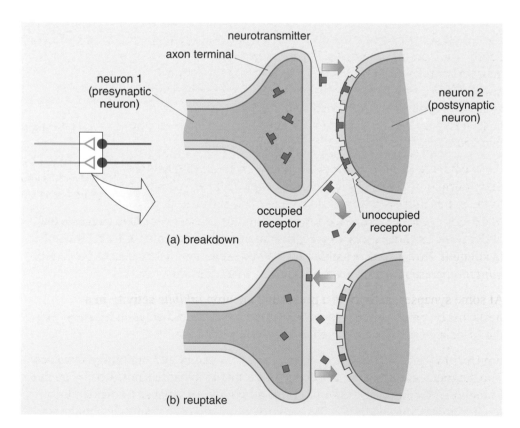

Figure 5.12 Inactivation of neurotransmitter: (a) by breakdown within the synapse and (b) by reuptake into the presynaptic neuron.

◆ Information is transmitted *between* neurons by which means?

◆ Chemical. (*Note*: some synapses do not follow this principle but they need not concern us here.)

As illustrated in Figure 5.13, the nervous system employs more than one type of neurotransmitter, labelled in this diagram as neurotransmitters A and B. Thus, for example, one synapse might employ glutamate as its neurotransmitter, whereas an immediately adjacent one might employ the different neurotransmitter, GABA. Glutamate is pronounced as glue-ter-mate. GABA is short for gamma-aminobutyric acid and is pronounced gab-er. Different neurotransmitters are shown in Figure 5.13 as forming different shapes. Correspondingly, there are different receptors in the two cases. So, even if a molecule of neurotransmitter A were to move across to the synapse employing neurotransmitter B, it would be ineffective since the shape does not fit the receptors for neurotransmitter B (Figure 5.13).

5.5.2 Excitation and inhibition at synapses

Earlier we described how action potentials in a presynaptic neuron (neuron 1 of Figure 5.11) cause the release of neurotransmitter that triggers activity in the form of action potentials in a postsynaptic neuron (neuron 2). In other words, at such synapses, neuron 1 *excites* neuron 2. The presynaptic neuron is described as 'excitatory' and the synapse between the two neurons is described as an **excitatory synapse**.

As you have seen, it is by means of one neuron exciting another that information (e.g. on tissue damage) gets from the periphery to the brain. However, as was noted at several stages in the book, it is not inevitable that a noxious stimulus causes pain. This suggests that, under some circumstances, nociceptive signals are blocked or at least reduced in strength. How is this possible? As well as excitation there is also a process of *inhibition* present. At the level of neurons, what does this mean?

At some synapses, activity in a presynaptic neuron *inhibits* activity in a postsynaptic neuron. Such a presynaptic neuron is described as 'inhibitory' and the associated synapse is termed an **inhibitory synapse**.

Figure 5.14 (overleaf) contrasts the action of excitatory and inhibitory synapses. The diagram shows neuron 1 making an excitatory synapse (indicated by an open triangle) with neuron 3. Neuron 2 forms an *inhibitory* synapse (indicated by a filled triangle) with neuron 3. The activity, if any, in each neuron is shown as a

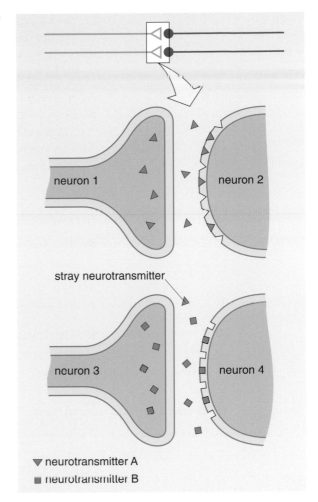

Figure 5.13 Schematic diagram of two different synapses employing two types of neurotransmitter, A and B.

Figure 5.14 Schematic diagram of excitatory (clear triangle) and inhibitory (filled triangle) synapses. (a) Inactivity; (b) neuron 1 active; (c) neurons 1 and 2 active; (d) increased inhibitory activity. Graphs show the frequency of action potentials in each neuron with time.

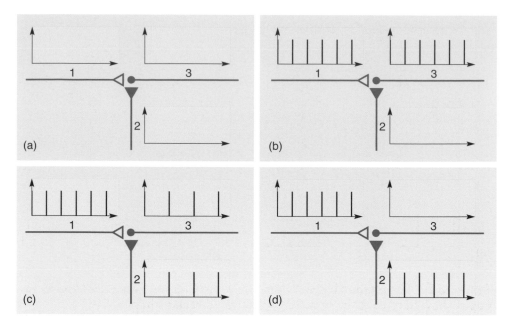

series of action potentials within the rectangles associated with each neuron. In Figure 5.14a there is no activity in any of the three neurons.

◆ With reference to Figure 5.14a, suppose that action potentials arise in neuron 1 (e.g. triggered by a stimulus at the neuron's sensory ending). What would be the effect on neuron 3?

◆ As is shown in Figure 5.14b, the result is the production of action potentials in neuron 3.

Suppose now that, with neuron 1 showing the same activity as in Figure 5.14b, the inhibitory neuron (neuron 2) shows a slight activity. As you can see, in Figure 5.14c, inhibition of the activity of neuron 3 consists of a reduced frequency of action potentials relative to Figure 5.14b.

◆ What would be the effect of increasing activity in neuron 2?

◆ Increased inhibition exerted on neuron 3, results in a further lowering of the frequency of action potentials (as shown in Figure 5.14d).

In other words, the activity of neuron 3 represents a 'balance' between competing signals that arrive via excitatory and inhibitory synapses. The enormous significance of excitation and inhibition will become apparent shortly, when the next chapter describes neurons and pain.

5.5.3 Manipulating synapses

The existence of natural chemical neurotransmitters in the nervous system offers the possibility of finding artificial chemical interventions to change events in the nervous system, e.g. to lower pain. People ingest, inhale or inject various chemicals in the implicit expectation that they will affect the brain. More specifically, these chemicals (such as alcohol and nicotine) affect the activity at billions of synapses in the nervous system.

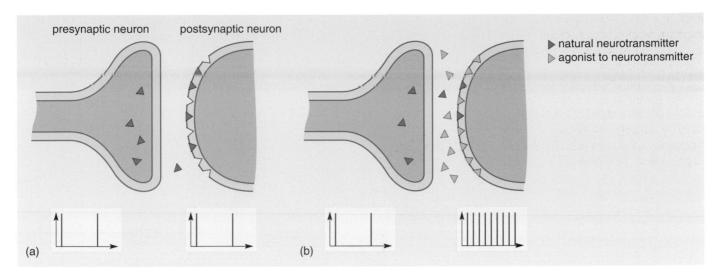

Figure 5.15 The relation between a natural neurotransmitter and its agonist. (a) without agonist; (b) with agonist. Graphs show the frequency of action potentials in each neuron.

Substances that occupy receptors at synapses and *mimic* the role of the natural neurotransmitter are termed **agonists**. This means that they produce the *same* effect on the postsynaptic neuron as the natural neurotransmitter (Figure 5.15).

Of particular interest in the context of pain, certain synapses in the CNS (central nervous system, i.e. the brain and spinal cord) employ chemical substances that belong to the group called **opioids** (oh-pee-oydz). One type of opioid is termed 'endorphin'. This term is derived from *end*ogenous mor*phin*e-like substance, indicative of its similarity to morphine. (The term 'endogenous' means that the source of the substance is within the body itself.) Opioids play a natural role in reducing the level of pain. Injection of the drug morphine, an agonist to these substances, augments the role of the natural equivalents.

By contrast to agonists, there are other substances that occupy receptors but thereby *block* the effect of the natural neurotransmitter – these are termed **antagonists**.

5.6 Some details of the brain

Examination of the structures and working of the brain and its component cells, e.g. the types of neurons and systems of neurons involved, allows investigators to unravel what the brain does. An unambiguous description of the brain is necessary for being able to ask sensible questions concerning what different bits of the brain do and how they relate to pain.

5.6.1 The brain requires fuels

The cells of the brain, e.g. the neurons, require a supply of oxygen and glucose in order to function. In this regard, they are just like the 'general' cells of the body (Figure 4.1b). The blood supply is brought to the brain's neurons in the cerebral arteries, as shown in Figure 5.16 (overleaf). Waste products are carried away from the brain's neurons by blood in veins. If there is damage to an artery in the brain, as in a blood clot blocking it or breaking of a blood vessel (causing a

The term 'cerebral' means related to the head, or more specifically the brain.

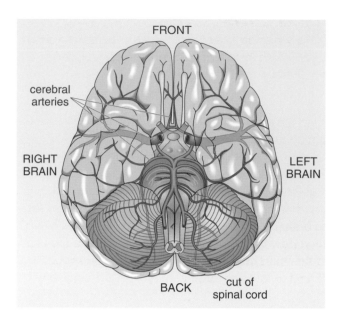

Figure 5.16 A view of the brain (from underneath) to reveal its arteries.

'stroke'), this can deny the neurons in the affected region their supply of nutrients. These neurons cannot function and will die. This can then disturb particular aspects of behaviour. For example, if the damage is to a specific region of the left side of the brain, there are often disturbances of speech, as can occur in stroke.

5.6.2 The hemispheres

Much of the brain can be divided into two halves, termed the **cerebral hemispheres**, left and right (often abbreviated as 'left brain' and 'right brain') (Figure 5.17). The diagrammatic convention employed in all anatomical drawings is that of the person whose body is being illustrated. Hence, in Figure 5.17 the left hemisphere is that to the person's left. You can also see that there are neurons that link the two hemispheres, forming the structure termed the 'corpus callosum'. By this means, information can be communicated from one cerebral hemisphere to the other.

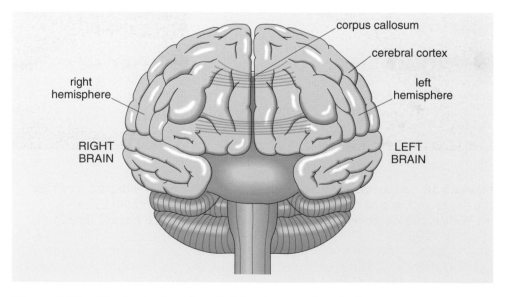

Figure 5.17 The brain showing division into two hemispheres.

The outer layer of the brain is termed the **cortex**, sometimes known as the 'cerebral cortex'. The cortex has a wrinkled appearance something like a walnut (Figure 5.17). There are a number of different techniques for observing and understanding the brain and two of these are described next.

5.6.3 Brain imaging

The techniques of **brain imaging** have developed very rapidly and are revolutionising the study of the brain (Figure 5.18). The production of action potentials by neurons requires energy (provided by glucose) and oxygen; the higher the frequency of action potentials, the higher the energy requirement. So, just as muscles that are highly active require relatively large amounts of fuel for energy, so do those parts of the brain that are particularly active. This is achieved by an automatic increase in blood flow to these parts. So, suppose that a noxious stimulus is applied. Regions of the brain involved with generating the sensation of pain (the 'pain matrix') will tend to become more active, with a diversion of blood to them.

If investigators can identify where the blood is going in large amounts, then they can identify the regions in which neurons are most active. In this way, they can locate the regions doing the most processing of information. Using one version of this imaging technique, investigators inject a radioactive tracer substance into the blood and then detect where it goes to in the brain. Figure 5.18b illustrates results obtained in this way.

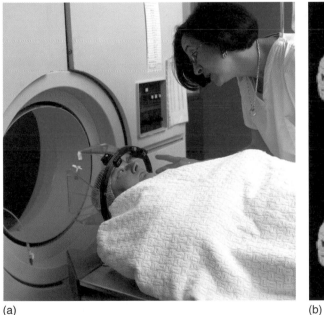
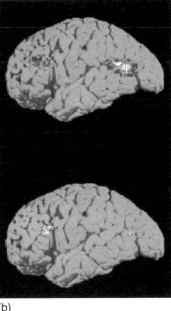

(a)   (b)

Figure 5.18   Brain imaging. (a) Apparatus; (b) images showing areas of high activity as yellow and red. (Photos: (a) CC Studio/Science Photo Library; (b) Wellcome Department of Cognitive Neurology/Science Photo Library)

5.6.4 Brain damage

Another source of information comes from looking at people with disruptions to a brain region. This can consist of a tumour, accidental damage, gunshot wounds or the result of a stroke. Surgical removal of diseased tissue can also be revealing. Damage to particular parts of the brain's pain matrix is associated with a reduction in that aspect of pain which is described as 'emotional disturbance'. By contrast, damage to other parts is associated with some loss of the sensory features of pain, e.g. where in the body the pain appears to arise.

Activity 5.2   The nervous system and synapses

Allow 30 minutes for this activity

Now would be an ideal time to study the interactive animation entitled 'The nervous system and synapses', which you will find on the DVD associated with this book. The animation presents the basics of the nervous system, including how synapses work. It will show how a simple reflex functions in terms of the neurons from which it is formed. There are interactive exercises designed to aid your understanding of what the terms 'excitation' and 'inhibition' mean, when applied to the links between neurons. The sequence also shows an animation of a chemical synapse.

If you are unable to complete this activity now, continue with the rest of the chapter and return to it as soon as you can.

5.7   The somatic and autonomic nervous systems

Researchers distinguish between the brain's influences on the body's external and internal environments. The external environment corresponds to the everyday sense of 'environment', consisting of such things as the weather, the buildings in which humans live and social companions, etc. The internal environment consists of all that is found inside the body, e.g. its temperature, the beating heart and the churning stomach, etc. The brain exerts an influence over both of these environments, as follows.

5.7.1 The somatic nervous system

The muscles that control the movements of the body, e.g. legs and arms, are termed 'skeletal muscles'. They derive this name from the fact that they attach to parts of the skeleton. The muscle shown in Figure 5.3b is of this kind.

The part of the nervous system that exerts control over the skeletal muscles is termed the **somatic nervous system (SNS)**. Acting via the SNS, humans are said to have 'voluntary control' over skeletal muscles. For example, you now have a free choice about closing this book and doing something else. Alternatively, if you are now still sitting and reading this book, this can equally be interpreted as the result of your voluntary choice, mediated via your cognition and the SNS!

In Figure 5.19, look at the pathway of neurons exemplified by neurons 1 and 2. These neurons project from the brain down the spinal cord to the skeletal muscles that control the position of the leg.

The term 'soma' means 'body'.

The term 'pathway' is sometimes used to describe the route taken by one or more neurons in linking two parts of the nervous system. It can also be used to describe the route taken by nerves consisting of many axons of neurons.

5.7.2 The autonomic nervous system

The branch of the nervous system that exerts an influence over the internal environment is termed the **autonomic nervous system** (abbreviated as **ANS**). The term 'autonomic', means 'self-governing'. This refers to the fact that, to some extent, it does its job autonomously, i.e. without conscious intervention by us. Temperature regulation, as in sweating and shivering (see Section 4.3 on homeostasis), exemplifies this.

The heart muscle, termed 'cardiac muscle', has an intrinsic tendency to contract in regular beats, i.e. even without an input from the nervous system. However, the rate of heart beats is increased or decreased by signals sent from particular regions of the brain, mediated via the ANS. Specifically, within the ANS, the control that the brain exerts is mediated via neurons exemplified by the sequence 3, 4 and 5 in Figure 5.19. Painful stimuli cause acceleration of heart rate.

◆ What will be an effect of such acceleration in so far as the muscles of the leg are concerned?

◆ An increased supply of blood, and thereby increased supply of glucose and oxygen, to the muscles.

◆ Can this be understood in terms of adaptive value?

◆ Pain could be a signal to take action as in fleeing or fighting. An acceleration of heart rate would be adaptive in facilitating such reactions, by increasing the 'fuel' supplied to the muscles.

Chapter 4 described another factor that increases heart rate and is released from an endocrine gland in response to such things as pain and threats.

◆ What is it?

◆ The hormone epinephrine, which is released from the suprarenal glands, and occupies receptors in the cardiac muscle.

Epinephrine is released by activity within the autonomic nervous system triggering the suprarenal glands to release the hormone into the bloodstream.

As another example of the role of the ANS, Figure 5.20 shows a cross-section through part of a blood vessel. In the wall, you can see the location of muscles, termed 'smooth muscles'. The ANS controls the degree of contraction of these muscles and hence the diameter of the vessel, which contributes to the control over blood flow. The term 'lumen' refers to the open channel of the tube.

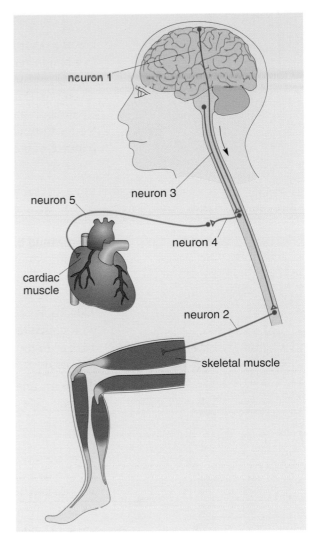

Figure 5.19 Neurons involved in control of the leg and heart muscles.

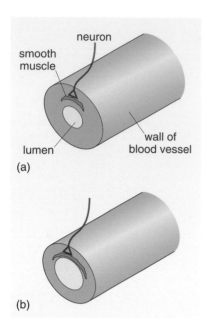

Figure 5.20 Cross-section through a blood vessel. (a) Muscle constricted and small diameter of vessel; (b) muscle relaxed and large diameter of vessel.

5.7.3 Coordination

Acting via the SNS and the ANS and in serving an adaptive role, the brain normally exerts a coordinated influence over the internal and external environments. For example, a time of relaxation is a good one for digestion of food to proceed, mediated via neurons that project from brain to gut. This involves an increase in the flow of blood to the gut. By contrast, a time of danger, as, for example, signalled by a sudden painful stimulus, is a time to suspend digestion temporarily. Thereby, more blood can flow to the skeletal muscles for 'fight or flight'.

For another example of coordination, suppose that you suddenly confront an angry bull and 'decide' to try your luck in running across the field to the fence. The SNS controls the activity of the skeletal muscles of the legs and thereby the movements of the legs. At the same time, the ANS also makes adjustments to activities inside the body in such a way that escape is facilitated. For example, heart rate is accelerated. This means an increased flow of blood is available to the skeletal muscles, since exertion requires increased levels of glucose and oxygen. The blood vessels supplying the skeletal muscles widen ('dilate') (Figure 5.20), which facilitates an increased blood flow to these muscles. Digestion is put on hold and blood is diverted away from the gut.

So, having introduced some general principles of the nervous system, the book now concentrates on the specifics of pain.

Summary of Chapter 5

5.1 Nerves are formed from bundles of the axons of neurons. Each axon is dedicated to convey a specific type of information. Some sensory information carried in axons is termed 'nociceptive'.

5.2 The brain and spinal cord constitute the central nervous system (CNS).

5.3 Sensory neurons convey information from the periphery of the body to the CNS and motor neurons convey information from the CNS to the muscles.

5.4 Information is carried within tracts (bundles of axons) in the spinal cord, to and from the brain.

5.5 A reflex is a fast and automatic reaction to a particular stimulus.

5.6 Neurons convey information by means of the frequency of action potentials in their axons.

5.7 A point of near contact between a neuron and another cell is termed a synapse.

5.8 At a synapse between two neurons, neurotransmitter is released from the presynaptic neuron and occupies receptors at the postsynaptic neuron.

5.9 Some synapses are excitatory and others are inhibitory.

5.10 Activity at synapses can be altered by agonists and antagonists to the natural neurotransmitter.

5.11 Acting by means of skeletal muscles, the somatic nervous system produces action on the external world in the form of behaviour.

5.12 Acting by means of smooth muscles and cardiac muscle, the autonomic nervous system controls the internal environment.

Learning outcomes for Chapter 5

After studying this chapter and its associated activities, you should be able to:

LO 5.1 Define and use, or recognise definitions and applications of, each of the terms printed in **bold** in the text. (Questions 5.1 to 5.5)

LO 5.2 Describe the relationship between the terms 'axon', 'neuron', 'synapse', 'tract' and 'nerve'. (Questions 5.1, 5.2 and 5.3)

LO 5.3 Distinguish between the meaning of the terms 'sensory neuron', 'interneuron' and 'motor neuron'. (Questions 5.1, 5.2 and 5.5 and DVD Activity 5.2)

LO 5.4 Describe the role that some neurons serve (i) in forming reflexes and (ii) in conveying information to and from the brain. (Question 5.4 and DVD Activity 5.2)

LO 5.5 Explain how information is transmitted along axons by means of action potentials. (Question 5.4 and DVD Activity 5.2)

LO 5.6 Describe the sequence of events at a synapse and some of the factors that can alter the transmission of information from one neuron to another. (Questions 5.3, 5.4 and 5.5)

LO 5.7 Give examples of how coordinated action involves cooperation between the somatic and autonomic nervous systems. (Question 5.5)

LO 5.8 Construct and interpret a graph showing data points. (Activity 5.1)

Self-assessment questions for Chapter 5

You had the opportunity to demonstrate LO 5.8 by completing Activity 5.1 and LOs 5.3, 5.4 and 5.5 by completing Activity 5.2 on the DVD.

Question 5.1 (LOs 5.1, 5.2 and 5.3)

With regard to Figure 5.3, suppose that the spinal cord in (a) were to suffer a complete break at the location indicated by the slice shown in (b). What effect would this have on sensation and the control of muscles?

Question 5.2 (LOs 5.1, 5.2 and 5.3)

Of the neurons numbered 1–4 in Figure 5.3b, which have axons that form part of (i) a nerve, (ii) a tract?

Question 5.3 (LOs 5.1, 5.2 and 5.6)

If a synapse is said to 'employ the neurotransmitter glutamate', what does this tell you about the presynaptic and postsynaptic neurons that almost come together at the synapse?

Question 5.4 (LOs 5.1, 5.4, 5.5 and 5.6)

In Figure 5.14b, suppose that an agonist to the neurotransmitter employed by neuron 2 is injected. What would be the expected effect on neuron 3?

Question 5.5 (LOs 5.1, 5.3, 5.6 and 5.7)

What would be the expected effect of injecting an agonist (i) to the neurotransmitter employed by nociceptive neurons and (ii) to epinephrine (in so far as the heart is concerned)? (*Note*: Agonists act at receptors to hormones just as they do at receptors to neurotransmitters.)

6 A FOCUS ON PAIN AND THE NERVOUS SYSTEM

This chapter will illustrate how an examination of the properties of neurons and the connections that they form enables some understanding of pain. We start by reiterating one of the book's central themes: although noxious stimuli can trigger pain, there is not a simple one-to-one link between the magnitude of the stimulus and the experience of pain. The organising theme of Chapter 6 is an attempt to explain this aspect of pain in terms of the properties of neurons. Based on this well-recognised variability in the link between stimulus and pain, the chapter identifies neural processes that trigger pain and other neural processes that inhibit activity in nociceptive pathways.

Since pain has been traditionally studied in terms of triggering by noxious stimuli, such pain forms the foundation of the account given here.

Figure 6.1 shows a pathway that transmits nociceptive information from the periphery of the body, via the spinal cord to various regions in the brain. These brain regions (and others not shown) considered together constitute the pain matrix. This chapter will look first at the peripheral part, then the spinal cord, and finally consider the brain processes that are involved in pain, such as the thalamus and regions of the cortex.

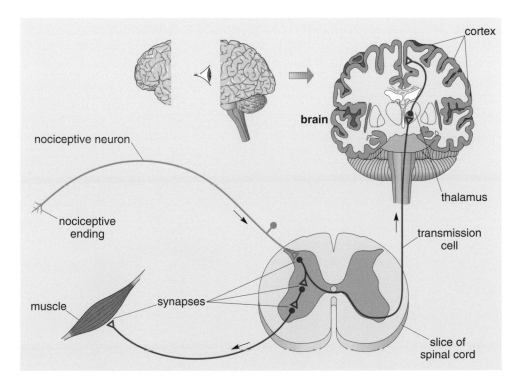

Figure 6.1 Pathway of nociceptive information. The brain section is shown in the small figure and enlarged in the large (based on Craig, 2003). The pathway shown is only one amongst several that transmit nociceptive information (Melzack and Wall, 1988).

6.1   The periphery

The nociceptive endings of the axons of nociceptive neurons are located throughout most regions of the body.

◆   What is the implication of this for pain?

◆   Tissue damage in most regions is associated with pain.

Interestingly, the brain itself does not contain any such nociceptive neurons. This means that brain surgery can be carried out on conscious patients (though, of course, the adjacent skin and other tissue is numbed with anaesthetic).

The expression **threshold of excitation** describes the level of intensity of stimulation (e.g. pressure applied to the sensory ending) at which a neuron first starts to be activated. This threshold depends upon the *diameter* of the axon. (If you cut through an axon, the diameter would be the width of the cut surface viewed 'end on'; see Figure 6.2.) The axons of nociceptive neurons have relatively small diameters compared with other sensory neurons. The diameter of an axon determines how much stimulation is required at the sensory ending before the threshold of excitation is exceeded and the neuron generates a train of action potentials. This can be illustrated by a graph (Figure 6.2) in which the amount of pressure being applied to the sensory ending of the axon appears along the horizontal axis and the frequency of action potentials is plotted on the vertical axis. Figure 6.2a shows the response of a nociceptive neuron to increasing pressure. The line representing the frequency of action potentials quickly increases from the point at which the pressure exceeds the threshold of excitation for this neuron (labelled T_S, to denote the threshold for a *small*-diameter axon).

Figure 6.2b shows the response of a neuron with a *large*-diameter axon (threshold of excitation = T_L), which is sensitive to harmless touch. Compare the response of these two neurons to pressure that starts from zero and increases steadily along the horizontal axis of the graphs.

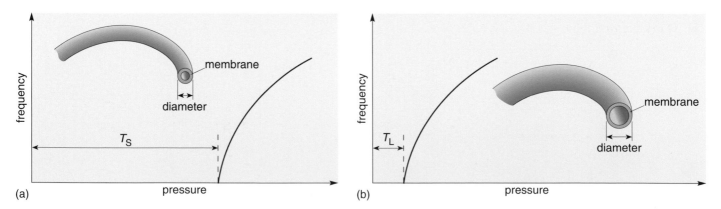

Figure 6.2   The response of neurons (in terms of action potentials) to pressure, showing the threshold of excitation (*T*). (a) Nociceptive neuron (having an axon of small diameter) and (b) neuron with a large-diameter axon.

◆ What *difference* do you see?

◆ Nociceptive neurons have a relatively high threshold of excitation (T_S), meaning only intense pressure will activate them (the line representing the frequency of action potentials begins to rise only at a point far along the 'pressure' axis). The neuron with a large-diameter axon has a much lower threshold (T_L) and begins generating action potentials when the pressure is slightly above zero.

The pressure sufficient to excite the nociceptive neurons would normally trigger pain, whereas the neurons with large-diameter axons are responsive to even harmless gentle pressure. The axons of both types of sensory neuron then convey the information about pressure to the CNS.

Different types of tissue damage can trigger activity in nociceptive neurons. These neurons can be activated by physical damage to the nociceptive ending itself. In addition, when cells in the neighbourhood of the nociceptive ending are damaged, the membranes of the neighbouring cells get broken and substances are released from the damaged cells. Some of these substances are able to activate nociceptive neurons at their axon endings or contribute towards their activation. A class of substance termed *prostaglandins* is released from damaged cells and they 'sensitise' the nociceptive endings (Figure 6.3).

◆ Compare Figures 6.3a and b. What effect do prostaglandins have on the threshold of excitation of the neuron?

◆ It is lowered by the action of prostaglandins, i.e. the neuron begins to generate action potentials at a *lower* pressure threshold.

Now look at Figures 6.4a and b, overleaf. Imagine that an amount of pressure (labelled P_X) is applied to the nociceptive neuron in both situations.

◆ What is the effect of prostaglandins on the frequency of action potentials produced in Figure 6.4b?

◆ It is increased relative to Figure 6.4a.

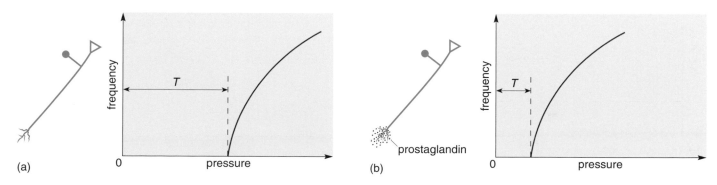

(a)　(b)

Figure 6.3　Responses of a nociceptive neuron to potentially damaging pressure, highlighting the difference in threshold T. (a) Without and (b) with sensitisation by prostaglandins.

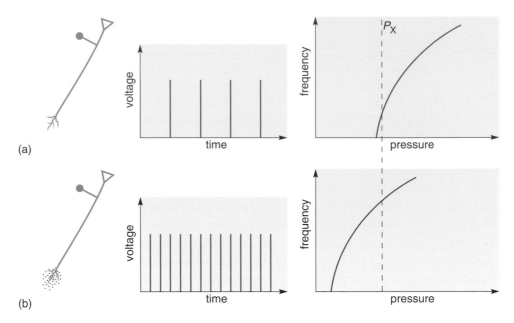

Figure 6.4   Responses of a nociceptive neuron to a sharp object, highlighting the result at an intensity of stimulation P_X. (a) Without and (b) with sensitisation by prostaglandins.

Action potentials travel along the axon to the axon terminal within the spinal cord, where they trigger the release of neurotransmitter.

6.2   The spinal cord

Within the spinal cord, nociceptive neurons (having small-diameter axons) make synaptic contact with other neurons (Figure 6.1). They tend to excite these second neurons in the sequence, a type of interneuron termed 'transmission cells', which then transmit action potentials to the brain region known as the thalamus (Figure 6.1). Nociceptive neurons are known to release two excitatory neurotransmitters: glutamate (which you met earlier) and 'substance P'.

A given amount of activity in a nociceptive neuron can trigger very different amounts of activity in a transmission cell. The variation depends upon events occurring around the synapse that forms the link between these two types of cell.

◆   What aspect of pain does this explain?

◆   A given amount of tissue damage can be associated with very different reported intensities of pain.

Some speak of 'gate control theory' rather than 'gate theory' but the terms mean the same.

This variability has become assimilated into a highly influential theory of pain, **gate theory**, proposed by Patrick Wall of University College, London and Ronald Melzack of McGill University, Canada. In this analogy, it is *as if* there is a gate at the spinal cord. When the gate is open, the nociceptive message can pass through but, when the gate is fully closed, the message gets no further than the axon terminal of the nociceptive neuron in the spinal cord. The gate can be at various degrees of open or shut. The term 'gate' is merely a useful metaphor; of course, there is not *literally* something that is raised and lowered or which swings on hinges but, none the less, a process that opens and closes the nociceptive pathway exists.

So what opens and closes the gate? According to the theory, there are two inputs to synapses that can do this:

1   Large-diameter axons with sensory endings at around the same location in the body as the endings of nociceptive neurons.

2   Axons that descend from the brain forming descending pathways.

For example, see Figure 6.5. Inputs to synapses 1 and 2 both oppose the tendency of nociceptive neurons to activate the transmission cells. The input to synapse 1 explains why gentle rubbing of the skin can reduce pain. For example, this is why you tend to rub a sore site such as a mosquito bite or eyes irritated by hay fever. Rubbing triggers activity in large-diameter axons, which have a low threshold of excitation, and this tends to oppose the transmission of the nociceptive signal arising from the same area. Such rubbing is not sufficient to trigger the higher-threshold nociceptive neurons.

The input to synapse 2 suggests a neural explanation of how, at least in part, cognitive factors such as expectations and shifts of attention might reduce pain. That is to say, the descending input provides a neural explanation for how techniques of cognitive therapy for pain might work.

Of course, Figure 6.5 is a gross simplification. It is designed simply to illustrate only certain features of pain. In reality, the connections among neurons are much more complex than this. Such complexity explains the different qualities of pain such as itching and burning.

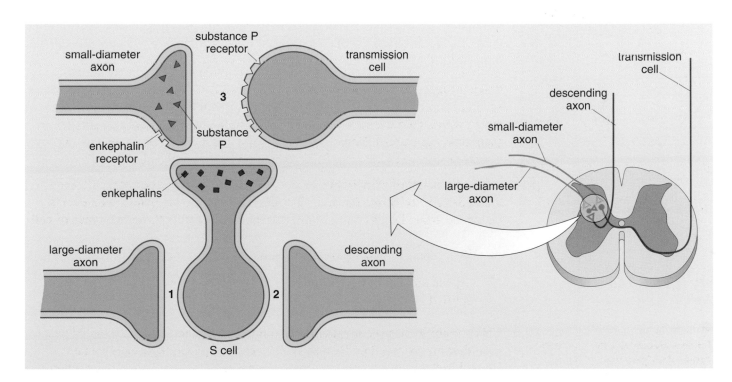

Figure 6.5   Junction of a small-diameter axon and a transmission cell in the spinal cord, showing how the gate is influenced by inputs from the skin (large-diameter axon) and the brain (descending axon). *Note:* for clarity some neurotransmitters and receptors have been omitted.

Look again at Figure 6.5. In the spinal cord, neurons with large-diameter axons as well as those axons descending from the brain, form excitatory synapses (1 and 2) upon a short neuron that is labelled 'S cell' (S stands for 'short'). When the S cell is excited by either or both of these routes, it releases a type of opioid termed *enkephalins*.

◆ What does 'being excited' mean?

◆ The S cell generates action potentials.

After release, enkephalins occupy enkephalin receptors.

◆ Where are these receptors in Figure 6.5?

◆ At the terminal of the small-diameter axon and at the region of the postsynaptic neuron (the transmission cell) that is just across the synapse.

Occupation of receptors at the terminal of the small-diameter axon reduces the amount of neurotransmitter, e.g. substance P, which is released. Occupation of receptors on the transmission cell *opposes* ('inhibits') the ability of the nociceptive neuron to excite the transmission cell at synapse 3. Both of these effects *reduce* the transmission of nociceptive information to the brain. Injection of opioid agonists at this site has a pain-reducing effect, whereas opioid antagonists increase pain.

Gate theory could provide a rationale for how certain individuals can suffer tissue damage in, for example, a sporting activity or a religious cause, with apparently rather little pain (Figure 6.6). They appear to have found the right behaviour or 'mind-set' to trigger the descending pathway.

6.3 The brain

If you look back to Figure 6.1, you can trace the route followed by nociceptive information carried by neurons from the periphery, up the spinal cord, and then in the brain. Note the neurons that project their axons from the thalamus to the cortex. Some of the neurons of the cortex are responsible for the sensory dimension of pain, i.e. discriminating the *location* in the body that is its source, and its *quality* as, say, tickling or burning. Other neurons are responsible for the *affective quality* of pain – its nastiness – a property you saw mentioned in Table 3.1.

Concerning the descending axons (Figure 6.5), these originate within the brain. They are excited by activity within various regions of the brain that concern attention and emotion. Psychological techniques such as distraction (described in the next chapter) are thought to involve triggering activity in these descending axons.

You have already met nociceptive and psychogenic pain. Now another type of pain can be introduced. The term **neurogenic pain** describes pain that arises from damage to neurons in either the CNS or the periphery. For example, if nociceptive neurons get damaged or squeezed, this can initiate the production

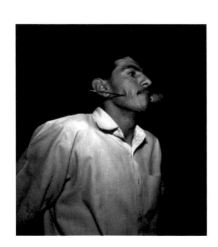

Figure 6.6 Stoical acceptance of physical injury in a religious cause by a member of the Rufias sect in Erbil, Iraq. (Photo: Sedat Aral/Rex Features)

of action potentials even in the absence of the normal noxious stimulus at their nociceptive endings. The result can be chronic intractable pain of a type that is described in a later activity (Activity 7.1). Now try Activity 6.1.

Activity 6.1a   Understanding gate theory
Activity 6.1b   The value of gate theory

Allow about 30 minutes

Now would be an ideal time to study the activities entitled 'Understanding gate theory' and 'The value of gate theory', which you will find on the DVD that accompanies this book. The first sequence uses animations to reinforce your understanding of the nervous system and pain, including the principles of gate theory. The second sequence, a video, shows interviews with pain therapists in which they discuss the value of gate theory in treating pain.

If you are unable to complete these activities now, continue with the rest of the chapter and return to them as soon as you can.

6.4   Anomalies of pain

The lack of a close association between tissue damage at a particular location and pain associated with the location has been described. Certain anomalies of pain exemplify further this lack of close association. Such phenomena make better sense if you understand how neurons connect together in the production of pain.

6.4.1   Plasticity and pain

Over time, pains can change in intensity. For example, following tissue damage, the intensity of pain can get worse over weeks. This points to changes that occur in the nervous system processes that underlie pain. A general feature of the CNS is its **plasticity**. This refers to the fact that, looking at the connections between neurons, the nervous system is not a static structure. By analogy with the material called 'plastic', these connections can change their structure (be 'moulded') as a result of various factors.

Synapses exhibit such plasticity of their structure and function. In Figure 6.7 (overleaf), neuron 1 forms an excitatory synapse on neuron 2. Figure 6.7a represents the original state of the synapse and Figure 6.7b represents the synapse after a change characterised as 'plasticity' has occurred. Assume that, in parts (a) and (b), the same level of activity occurs in neuron 1.

◆   Compare the response of neuron 2 between parts (a) and (b). What is the difference in the sensitivity of neuron 2 to activity in neuron 1?

◆   The sensitivity in (b) has increased relative to (a). There is increased postsynaptic activity in (b) as compared with (a), i.e. a higher frequency of action potentials in neuron 2 in (b).

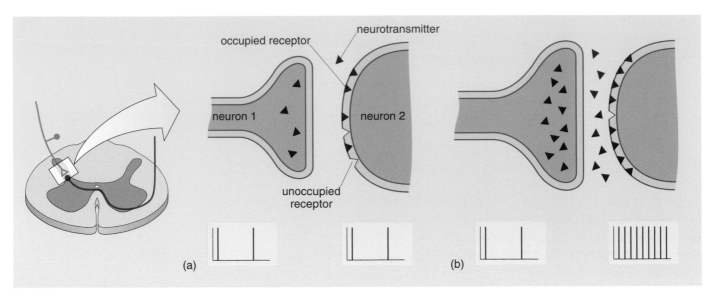

Figure 6.7 Plasticity at a synapse. (a) Start and (b) later. The graph to the right in each part shows activity in neuron 2 that is triggered by activity in neuron 1 (shown to the left).

Again, look carefully at Figure 6.7 and compare (a) and (b).

◆ What are the changes at the synapse that underlie the increased sensitivity?

◆ At the presynaptic neuron, the axon terminal has got bigger. There is (i) an increased area of release of neurotransmitter, which facilitates greater release of neurotransmitter, and (ii) at the postsynaptic neuron, there is an increased density of receptors.

The more neurotransmitter that is released, and the greater the number of receptors to which it attaches, the greater is the effect in terms of frequency of action potentials generated in neuron 2.

Plasticity is a very general property shown throughout the nervous system. So, what is the adaptive value of this property? What advantage does it bring? Think of learning a new skill. Underlying the changes in behaviour, corresponding changes occur in the connections within the nervous system. The control of muscles becomes more refined with experience. Plasticity clearly has adaptive value as a property of the nervous system underlying the capacity to modify behaviour, as in development and learning.

However, as you probably have realised, plasticity is something of a double-edged sword. It can be an unmitigated disaster in the context of pain, when neural connections underlying the production of pain also show plasticity, such that the pathway becomes sensitised. A much lower level of activity is then sufficient to start activation leading to pain, a feature of neurogenic pain. This is thought to underlie some chronic pains (Sufka and Turner, 2005). Thus, what would normally be an acute pain has the potential to become a chronic pain (Roth, 2000). In pain research, such plasticity is termed **wind-up**. Figure 6.7 shows wind-up at a synapse in the spinal cord. Wind-up probably also occurs in the neurons of the pain matrix in the brain.

So, let us summarise wind-up in the context of adaptive value:

1   Plasticity is a broad general property exhibited throughout the nervous system.

2   As a general feature, plasticity has an overall adaptive value in permitting change in activity in the nervous system.

3   However, as a result of plasticity, the nociceptive pathway can become sensitised chronically.

4   Plasticity of parts of the CNS underlies the experience of chronic pain.

5   Chronic pain appears to serve no adaptive role.

From adaptive considerations, would it have been better if those regions underlying pain were unable to display plasticity? Indeed, it might well have been so! This again makes the point that evolution cannot arrive at the perfect solution. There are inevitable trade-offs between benefits and costs.

6.4.2 Phantom pain

Phantom sensations are commonly experienced 'in' body regions (e.g. limbs) that have been amputated, either surgically or in accidents. As many as 30% of women, who have had breast removal for cancer (mastectomy), experience phantom sensations 'in' the missing breast (Keefe et al., 2005). Amongst these sensations, patients frequently report very realistic pains, which appear to arise in the lost body part. This is termed **phantom pain**.

Evidence suggests that phantom pain arises from a number of interacting factors. Plasticity (Section 6.4.1), i.e. changes in the connections between neurons, is central to trying to understand it. To reiterate the message of the last section, the nervous system is not a *static* mosaic of connections but a system that reshapes itself as a result of what is experienced. Consider the body prior to damage and the pathways that originally projected from the particular (now) lost body region to the pain matrix in the brain. Following the loss, wind-up between neurons in what remains intact within these pathways appears to be a contributory factor to phantom pain (Sufka and Turner, 2005). When the normal input to a transmission cell (Figure 6.5) is disrupted as a result of loss of a body part, the transmission cell can become hypersensitive, such that it even generates action potentials *spontaneously* (Melzack and Wall, 1988). These are transmitted to the brain just as if they were triggered by a nociceptive input. Metaphorically speaking, the interconnected neurons 'take on a life of their own'.

In addition, now deprived of their normal inputs, transmission cells appear to send out chemical signals to other neurons (Figure 6.8, overleaf). These signals, in effect, invite the 'receiving neurons' to send out branches which form new synapses on the signalling cells. As a result of such newly formed connections, neurons that detect harmless events acquire the capacity to excite the transmission cells. Therefore, an otherwise gentle and innocuous touch of the skin can now trigger pain.

On being subjected to such input, the pain matrix in the brain also appears to show wind-up. It becomes hypersensitive with some capacity to generate activity

You may recall that in Activity 3.1 on the DVD, Brian gives an account of a phantom effect.

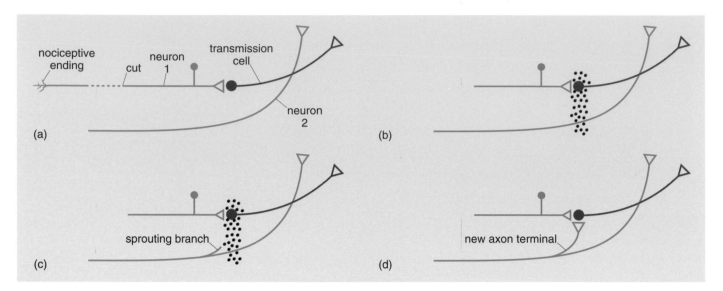

Figure 6.8 A possible sequence following loss of a body part. (a) Condition prior to loss and showing where cut occurs; (b) loss of body part and release of signalling chemical; (c) axon terminal of a nociceptive neuron degenerates due to loss of activity, and passing axon (axon 2) conveying innocuous information responds to the signal; (d) new synaptic contact is established.

on its own. Tragically, a consequence of this is that surgical intervention below the level of the brain to cut nociceptive pathways can then prove ineffective in reducing pain (Melzack and Wall, 1988).

Phantom pain is an example of a neurogenic pain.

◆ What is meant by this?

◆ Pain that cannot be accounted for by noxious stimulation but arises from abnormal neural activity occurring somewhere within the nociceptive pathway.

6.4.3 Referred pain

Sometimes pain due to tissue damage in one region of the body can be felt as arising in a different region, a phenomenon termed **referred pain**. The person feels pain apparently arising 'in' what is, in fact, a perfectly intact region of the body. For example, pain triggered by tissue damage in the heart can be 'referred to' the left shoulder and arm, where it is felt to arise. Pain arising from a stone in the kidney can be experienced as if originating in the genitals. Such referrals are not haphazard but follow certain patterns. Why do they occur?

It is because of the way that the nervous system is constructed. Figure 6.9 shows a convergence onto the same transmission cell of neural signals arising at the skin and at an internal organ. Presumably, people are used to interpreting messages arising from tissue damage at the skin as pain. When the same transmission cell is triggered by disruption at the internal organ, its activity is interpreted as pain arising at the skin.

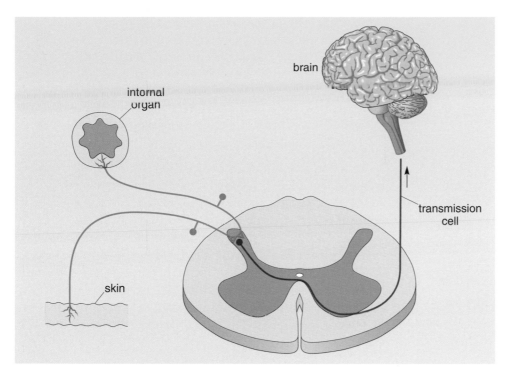

Figure 6.9 Part of the neural basis of referred pain.

In addition, as a result of the complex interconnections between neurons, an additional source of pain can appear. In association with the experience of referred pain arising from an organ, 'trigger points' on the skin are revealed, such that gentle stimulation of these areas of skin can trigger intense pain (Melzack and Wall, 1988).

This section has focused on nociceptive pain. Based on an understanding of this, researchers can speculate on the brain mechanisms that underlie psychogenic pain.

6.5   Relating nociceptive pain to psychogenic pain

Using imaging techniques, it is possible to examine the activity of brain regions of people, as they experience the presentation of noxious stimuli.

◆ How is this technique possible (recall Section 5.6.3)?

◆ Regions in which the neurons are particularly active have a relatively large flow of blood to them. A large flow implies a high neuronal activity and a high level of information processing.

Imaging techniques yield insight into not only nociceptive but also psychogenic pain (Figure 6.10, overleaf). How do investigators produce psychogenic triggers, so that they can examine which regions of the brain are activated? Do they take a normal day-to-day ('baseline') recording of a person's brain activity, wait in hope for the unfortunate soul to be jilted, and then quickly try to gain another recording? It might sound like a formidable task, if not entirely farcical. In reality, the human ego would appear to be so fragile that the experiment is easier than might be imagined.

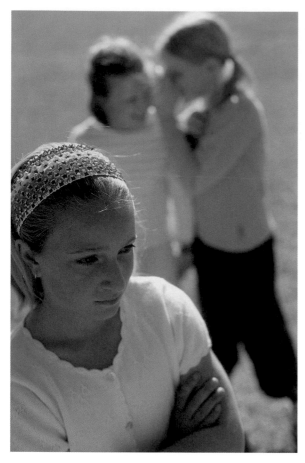

Figure 6.10 Can social rejection cause pain? Can there be a laboratory simulation of social rejection? (Photo: Photolibrary.com)

For example, participants in an experiment were asked to lie in a scanner and engage in a computerised game of 'virtual ball-tossing', while researchers produced images of the activity of their brains (Eisenberger et al., 2003). Although the participants imagined that they had a partner, in fact the moves of the 'partner' were programmed by computer. Suddenly, mid-game, it was announced to each participant that he (and, yes, they were male) had been excluded from the game.

On a scale of psychological distress, one would hardly have imagined that exclusion would rank as the most traumatic, alongside grief, being jilted or divorce. Indeed, with such obligations as looming deadlines, you might well have welcomed exclusion, having better things to do with your precious time than to lie with your head in a scanner playing virtual ball-tossing. However, for these participants, exclusion triggered activation in some of the same brain regions (e.g. parts of the cortex) as are activated by a noxious stimulus. So, in a real sense, social rejection appears to hurt and has a physical basis in the brain.

It is also possible to form images of the brain at work while someone feels empathy for the suffering of a person close to them (Singer et al., 2004). Using imaging techniques, women's brains were examined while their male partners were subjected to painful stimulation to the hand. Observing the partner in pain triggered parts of the pain matrix of the observer. That is, it seems the woman could literally *feel* something of her partner's pain.

Summary of Chapter 6

6.1 The term 'threshold of excitation' describes the level of stimulation needed to trigger activity in a neuron. It is relatively high in nociceptive neurons.

6.2 The gate theory suggests that, at the junction of nociceptive neurons and transmission cells in the spinal cord, there is, metaphorically speaking, a gate.

6.3 The gate can be closed by activity in (i) sensory neurons which have large-diameter axons and which project from the site of damage and (ii) axons descending from the brain.

6.4 Connections between neurons in the nociceptive pathway can exhibit plasticity, with a subsequent increase in pain, termed 'wind-up'.

6.5 The term 'phantom pain' refers to pain that appears to arise in a part of the body that no longer exists, e.g. an amputated limb.

6.6 The term 'referred pain' describes pain that appears to arise in an intact part of the body, whereas the real source is a disturbance at some other location.

6.7 Activation of some of the same regions of the brain (e.g. parts of the cortex) underlies the experience of nociceptive and psychogenic pain.

Learning outcomes for Chapter 6

After studying this chapter and its associated activities, you should be able to:

LO 6.1 Define and use, or recognise definitions and applications of, each of the terms printed in **bold** in the text. (Question 6.1 to 6.5)

LO 6.2 Describe what is meant by the term 'gate theory' and how gating can be understood in terms of the neurons involved. (Question 6.1 and DVD Activities 6.1a and 6.1b)

LO 6.3 Explain what is meant by the notion of 'plasticity' of the nervous system and relate this to pain. (Questions 6.2 and 6.3)

LO 6.4 Explain what is meant by 'phantom pain' and how it might arise. (Question 6.4)

LO 6.5 Describe how a knowledge of neural connections in the spinal cord can help the understanding of referred pain. (Question 6.5)

LO 6.6 Describe the evidence for the claim that the pains of social exclusion and empathy have a physical basis in the brain. (Question 6.2)

Self-assessment questions for Chapter 6

You also had the opportunity to demonstrate LO 6.2 by completing Activities 6.1a and 6.1b on the DVD.

Question 6.1 (LOs 6.1 and 6.2)

(a) The neuron that is labelled S in Figure 6.5 is one of which class: (i) sensory, (ii) motor or (iii) interneuron? (b) Suppose that someone is experiencing pain as a result of activation of the nociceptive neuron. However, some relief is being obtained since both the large-diameter axon and the descending axon are active. What would be the effect of an antagonist to the neurotransmitter employed by the S cell?

Question 6.2 (LOs 6.1, 6.3 and 6.6)

Suppose someone is able to reduce the pain of rejection by means of a conscious strategy of restating the problem in more positive terms. In Figure 3.4, the route represented by which arrow is being activated?

Question 6.3 (LOs 6.1 and 6.3)

Suppose that in Figure 6.7 the neurotransmitter shown is glutamate, which has an excitatory effect. Wind-up would be characterised by which of the following?

(i) Increased glutamate receptor density on the postsynaptic neuron.

(ii) Decreased glutamate receptor density on the postsynaptic neuron.

(iii) Increased release of glutamate from the presynaptic neuron for a given frequency of action potentials.

(iv) Decreased release of glutamate from the presynaptic neuron for a given frequency of action potentials.

Question 6.4 (LOs 6.1 and 6.4)

Suppose that a doctor writes on his/her notes 'phantom pain associated with wind-up'. What kind of report from the patient is most likely to be associated with this description?

Question 6.5 (LOs 6.1 and 6.5)

In Figure 6.9, the two synapses shown would be described as which of the following?

(i) excitatory

(ii) inhibitory

(iii) one excitatory and one inhibitory.

7 TREATING PAIN

Of course, the treatment of pain is of great personal, social, economic and ethical significance. Treatments vary from surgical, through electrical and chemical, to psychological therapies. These can be understood in terms of the pathways of neurons and brain regions involved in pain, as well as from a psychological perspective. This chapter describes types of treatment.

Although treatments differ in being biological (e.g. use of a drug) or psychological (e.g. counselling), any success that they have is bound to reflect changes in both the biology *and* psychology of the patient. That is, a psychobiological perspective would avoid dogma as to whether something works by means of changes that are *either* biological *or* psychological. This perspective gives a theoretical rationale for a pragmatic approach to therapy that exploits an array of treatments.

7.1 Chemical interventions

The term **analgesia** refers to a reduction in pain. Substances that reduce pain are known as **analgesics**.

In Chapter 5, Section 5.5.3, the substances termed 'agonist' and 'antagonist' were introduced.

◆ In principle, how might each of these classes of substance be used for the control of pain?

◆ Antagonists to the neurotransmitters in the nociceptive pathway might seem to be a type of intervention. Reciprocally, agonists to the neurotransmitters employed in regions of CNS that play a role in lowering pain are another possibility.

This section will describe some agonists and antagonists, as well as other chemical interventions for the control of pain.

You might feel that a place to start an investigation is with an antagonist to the neurotransmitters employed at the synapses between nociceptive neurons and transmission cells in the spinal cord. However, in practice, this would be problematic. The neurotransmitters (e.g. glutamate) employed at these synapses are found not only there but also play a wide variety of roles throughout the CNS. How would an antagonist specifically target the population of neurons involved in nociception? If a patient were to take a sufficient quantity of an antagonist to reduce pain, it might disrupt a range of activities, e.g. the control of balance or vision. Such undesired effects of a treatment are termed **side-effects**.

Figure 7.1a (overleaf) shows the normal transmission of nociceptive information from tissue damage at the periphery (the foot), to the spinal cord, and ascending in the spinal cord towards the brain. Figure 7.1b–d shows the effects of some well-established chemical interventions to block such transmission. We will discuss each in turn.

Figure 7.1 Effects of some analgesic substances. (a) no analgesic; (b) aspirin; (c) lignocaine injected in the vicinity of the length of axon between locations 2 and 3; (d) opiates. Graphs show the action potentials recorded at each of four sites between the periphery and the spinal cord (numbered 1, 2, 3 and 4).

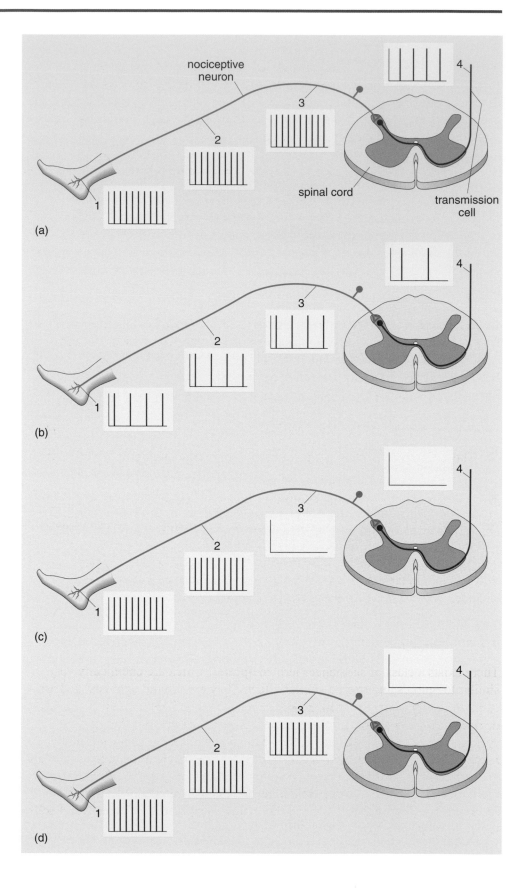

7.1.1 Aspirin

Aspirin is a form of mild analgesic, which works in the following way. Prostaglandins sensitise the sensory endings of nociceptive neurons and lower the threshold of excitation (Figures 6.3 and 6.4). Thereby, a relatively mild stimulus can trigger pain. Aspirin blocks the release of prostaglandins, and hence reduces the sensitivity of the nociceptive endings.

◆ What effect does this treatment have so far as action potentials are concerned (Figure 7.1a and b)?

◆ It reduces the frequency at which action potentials are initiated at the nociceptive ending (see location 1 and subsequent locations in Figure 7.1b as compared to part a).

7.1.2 Lignocaine

In dental surgery, you might have received a local injection of lignocaine. This chemical blocks the channels in the cell membrane through which ions pass (described in Chapter 5, Section 5.4). This movement of ions would normally form the basis of the action potential. Suppose that in Figure 7.1c, lignocaine is injected at a site between locations 2 and 3.

◆ What is the effect of lignocaine (Figure 7.1c)?

◆ The action potential cannot get past the site of the injection.

◆ Why do people feel numbness following the injection?

◆ Lignocaine does not discriminate between types of neuron and so blocks the ion channels in all the sensory and motor neurons in the region of the injection. For example, those neurons that normally convey messages on touch in the mouth would be equally affected as those that convey nociceptive information arising from having a tooth drilled.

7.1.3 Opiates

There exists a class of substances termed **opiates**, which are chemically very similar to opioids and exert a similar effect. They are 'opioid agonists' and are exemplified by morphine, which is taken for pain relief, and heroin. In the CNS, neurons that process nociceptive information contain receptors for opioids. At one such site (look back at Figure 6.5), opioids block the transmission of nociceptive signals at the spinal cord. Opioid receptors are at the axon terminals and are shown specifically as enkephalin receptors in Figure 6.5. Opiates target various sites in the CNS where opioid receptors are located and occupy these receptors. See Figure 7.1d for the result of their action in the spinal cord. Another location of opioid receptors is in the brain.

7.1.4 Antidepressants

Antidepressants are used in treating nociceptive pain. Their efficacy does not depend upon the patient suffering from depression, though, as noted, this can exacerbate pain. A factor in explaining the efficacy of certain antidepressants could be that they target synapses that employ the neurotransmitter termed serotonin. Serotonin is thought to act by changing the characteristics of neurons underlying emotion. Antidepressants block the reuptake of serotonin (Figure 5.12b).

◆ How does this affect transmission across the synapse?

◆ By blocking reuptake of serotonin, the amount of serotonin present in the synapse remains higher than normal. This increases the occupation of receptors at the postsynaptic membrane. Hence, the transmission sensitivity of the synapse is increased.

Serotonin seems to be implicated not only in brain processes that underlie the basis of depression (the normally intended target of antidepressants) but also acts as a neurotransmitter in the descending pathways that 'close the pain gate' (Caraceni et al., 2000).

An effect of the herbal remedy, St John's Wort, in lowering pain has been reported (Müller et al., 2004). This herb has effects at synapses that employ serotonin. The authors did not suggest that this herb is a panacea but it is one more weapon in the armoury of possible treatments.

7.1.6 Cultural, social and legal dimensions

Use of drugs occurs within a culture, which prescribes certain customs and laws governing their use and outlaws other uses. Apart from professional prescription by doctors, drugs can be recommended by friends, dealers or healers of various kinds.

In the Andes of South America, leaves of the coca plant are chewed for their mood-enhancing and energy-boosting properties, as well as to counter pain (Figure 7.2). They affect neurotransmission at particular classes of synapse in the CNS. A derivative of the coca plant, cocaine also has a long history of use as both psychological prop and analgesic. Indeed, cocaine could be purchased over the counter in England until around 1916. A famous user was Sigmund Freud, the Viennese pioneer of psychoanalysis, who took it as both mood-enhancer and analgesic (Clark, 1980).

The class of drug derived from the opium poppy has a long history as both mood-enhancer and analgesic. In the 1600s, opium was in common use in England as a treatment for pain (ABPI, 2007). As was noted earlier, opiates such as heroin have their natural equivalents in the body, as does cannabis, another class of drug.

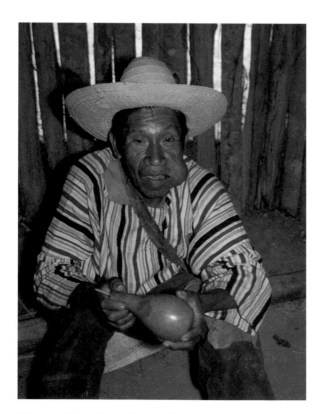

Figure 7.2 Coca leaves have been chewed by people in the Andes for over a thousand years. What effect do they have? (Photo: Eye Ubiquitous/Rex Features)

The use of cannabis for the relief of chronic pain can be traced back thousands of years, the earliest records being from China (Russo, 1998). Historically, various drugs have fallen in and out of official favour. On falling out, the drug's use sometimes continues unofficially and illegally. Cannabis exemplifies this. These days, few are aware of the importance that cannabis-based drugs once held in Western medicine. Now, presumably as a result of the drug's association with 1960s 'wild living', its name evokes images of pleasure rather than pain relief and it is illegal or highly restricted and street cannabis is associated with certain serious health risks. However, a survey carried out in Nova Scotia, Canada, revealed pain relief to be a common medicinal use of cannabis (Ware et al., 2003). Spurred by anecdotal evidence, the medical profession is now taking tentative steps to reinvestigate this use.

Also, in some countries excessive alcohol intake, particularly in elderly people, serves as medication for chronic pain. Brennan et al. (2005) found this amongst Californians.

All the drugs described in this section target receptors in the brain and have effects on both mood and pain. Cannabis and opium have natural equivalents produced by the body (enkephalins, a form of opioid, were described in Chapter 6). This suggests that, in the case of cannabis, as with opium, the drug-form mimics the action of a natural substance (Box 7.1).

Box 7.1 (Enrichment) Addiction

That some of the drugs used to treat pain are either identical or nearly identical to those that are the source of addiction is of considerable social relevance. Some doctors are reluctant to prescribe opiates for pain on the grounds that, after recovery, the patient might display an addiction to them. This is most unfortunate because in reality, there is only a slight danger of addiction following their use for pain relief (Melzack, 1988). The person seeking 'street drugs' usually wants them as a crutch for psychogenic pain and it is very rare that someone not in such distress develops an addiction.

 If you are studying this book as part of an Open University course, this would be a good point to try Activities C1 and C2 described in the *Companion* text.

7.2 Transcutaneous electrical nerve stimulation

Gate theory suggested that activity within the large-diameter axons of a type of sensory neuron could oppose the ability of nociceptive neurons to excite transmission cells, i.e. to 'close the gate'.

◆ What would be the effect of artificial stimulation of large-diameter axons in a region of skin triggering the pain?

◆ This would be expected to lower the pain.

This consideration led to the development of the therapeutic technique termed **transcutaneous electrical nerve stimulation** (TENS). TENS machines are now for sale over the counter in many wealthier parts of the world. TENS involves

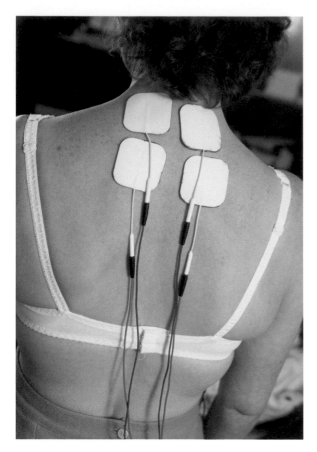

Figure 7.3 Patient using TENS machine (Photo: Science Photo Library)

applying weak electrical stimulation at the skin corresponding to an affected area (Figure 7.3).

◆ What is a factor limiting the intensity of stimulation applied?

◆ If it were too high, it might excite high-threshold nociceptive neurons as well as the lower-threshold neurons with axons of larger diameter. Pain would then be made worse.

7.3   Surgical intervention

Figure 6.1 showed the route followed by nociceptive information from the periphery to the brain. Surgical intervention within the route, to sever the neural pathways, might appear to be a viable intervention for the most chronic and intractable pains. Such intervention might seem straightforward but it is beset with problems. Pathways carrying nociceptive information are surrounded by others that carry information on harmless events. Inevitably, the lesion would also damage pathways carrying non-pain-related information and therefore cause some functional impairment.

Alas, often the pain reappears following the surgery, as if coming from the same bodily site as before. So, the results have been somewhat disappointing and this reinforces the important message about pain, which forms an over-arching theme of this book, as follows.

Pain can be associated with specific activity in particular sensory pathways. However, the brain systems underlying pain can sometimes 'take on a life of their own'. This means that, even if the sensory input is cut, the brain mechanisms, the 'pain matrix', can sometimes show spontaneous activity, in part reflecting wind-up.

7.4   Psychological intervention

7.4.1 Underlying principles

Gate theory provides a valuable rationale for psychological interventions to alleviate pain. Psychological effects arising in the brain are able to block the transmission of nociceptive information.

◆ How would gate theory explain this?

◆ A pathway descends from the brain to a gate in the nociceptive pathway and this provides one mechanism whereby psychological factors can block incoming information (i.e. 'close the gate').

Gate theory helps to bring together biological and psychological understanding of pain therapy. A psychological factor that plays an important role in the reaction to a noxious stimulus is whether patients perceive that they have *control* over the situation (Salomons et al., 2004). Psychological techniques attempt to give patients control and understanding of their possession of such control.

In one experiment, participants were told that they had control over a noxious stimulus by means of a joystick lever. In the so-called 'controllable condition', by responding on the lever, they could reduce the strength of the noxious stimulus. In fact, the lever was without effect and so the participants were duped. In the 'uncontrollable condition', participants were given exactly the same access to a lever and asked to respond but were instructed that their actions would be without effect on the noxious stimulus. Thus, the amount of noxious stimulation was identical in the two conditions, which differed only in the participants' *perception* of controllability.

Participants' brains were imaged during the experiment. Regions of the pain matrix (e.g. particular regions of the cerebral cortex) were activated under both conditions but were more strongly activated in the 'uncontrollable' condition. So, according to a biological measure, brain activity, belief in the controllability of pain reduces its intensity.

7.4.2 Cognitive-behavioural factors and therapy

Patients who score high on a questionnaire that measures *helplessness* tend to report high levels of pain and psychological distress in response to a given pain-eliciting condition (Keefe et al., 2005). Some researchers suggest that there is a 'pain-stress cycle', in which pain and stress form a vicious cycle (Gatchel and Weisberg, 2000).

◆ What could be meant by this?

◆ Pain increases stress and this in turn amplifies pain, which creates further stress, and so on.

Conversely, in response to the same triggers to pain, those patients who have a high measure of *self-efficacy* (i.e. a feeling of being able to control events) report lower levels of pain.

◆ Does this *prove* that psychological factors produce changes in pain level?

◆ No. Further information is needed before cause and effect can be teased apart. At least in principle, it could be that the psychological factors depend upon levels of pain, e.g. patients having the most pain are caused to feel helpless as a result.

However, experimentation has shown that, when psychological factors are manipulated, changes in pain often follow this, pointing to a causal role of psychological factors ('cognition') in pain.

So-called 'cognitive-behavioural models' are based on the observation that beliefs and expectations concerning pain play a role in how pain is perceived and how well people adjust to it. Therapy that is based on such ideas, termed **cognitive-behavioural therapy** (CBT), is designed to create feelings of coping and self-efficacy (Keefe et al., 2005). Patients are taught how to challenge negative thoughts that accompany pain and how to undermine 'catastrophising thoughts' (e.g. 'life is hopeless and I am helpless'). They are taught how to divert attention from pain and to create affectively positive images, to imagine positive scenes.

For example, consider a study of people with non-cardiac chest pain, who received a cognitive-behavioural intervention. When the patients were able to reattribute the cause of their pain to 'stress', there was a reduction in reported chest pain (Looper et al., 2002).

7.4.3 Hypnosis

Hypnosis can be defined as 'a social interaction in which one person, designated the subject, responds to suggestions offered by another person, designated the hypnotist, for experiences involving alterations in perception, memory and voluntary action' (Kihstrom, cited by Patterson, 2004). Some theorists believe that people enter an altered and unique state of consciousness when hypnotised (Patterson, 2004).

The hypnotherapist can attempt to alter the pain patient's tendency to catastrophise the situation. A reduction in pain level can sometimes be achieved by hypnosis. Sometimes a strange effect is seen under hypnosis, as follows. The physiological indicators of pain, such as heart rate, show an unchanged reaction to the nociceptive stimulus, whereas the patient's conscious report indicates a reduction in pain (Melzack and Wall, 1988).

Now see Box 7.2.

Box 7.2 (Enrichment) A reflection on analgesia in the human zoo

Techniques, such as injecting opiates for analgesia, involve a sophisticated modern technology: production of hypodermic syringes and extraction and refinement of the drug from poppy plants. Similarly, transcutaneous electrical nerve stimulation involves an apparatus for the application of electric currents to a site that is triggering pain. These techniques are the products of life in a modern technological society. Yet they seem to exploit processes that appeared early in evolution, as means of countering pain. Opiates tap into a natural analgesic process involving particular systems of neurons (Figure 6.5). Similarly, the electrical stimulation of large-diameter axons involves a system that would naturally be activated by rubbing the skin. So, it appears that evolution has produced not only a pain system but a natural system of analgesia. Of course, evolutionary processes did not produce these neural systems, only to leave them waiting millions of years for an industrial society to develop the means to exploit them! By now, if not sooner, you might be puzzled and be asking two related questions.

- If pain has adaptive value, what could be the adaptive value of a natural analgesic system that counters pain?

- What natural situations would tend to trigger the analgesic processes?

This is the cue for speculation, as follows. Consider first the descending pathways that help to block nociceptive signals. Pain is of general adaptive value but there might be occasions when it is temporarily to an animal's advantage to block the nociceptive signal, for example, when running injured from a predator. That is to say, injury occurs but pain is suppressed or lowered. Only when reaching safety, might it be to the animal's advantage to react to pain, as in limiting movement and resting (recall Figure 3.2). The descending pathway could be triggered naturally by the assessment of the need to escape. Opiates and psychological interventions to counter pain appear to work by means of tapping into this process of natural analgesia.

Consider now the advantage of a system of pain inhibition that involves the activation of large-diameter axons. One possibility is that this encourages an animal to lick wounds since it lowers pain. Such licking could promote wound healing. In these terms, the TENS machine exploits part of this process by activating large-diameter axons.

The next chapter will discuss a further factor that needs to be taken into account in any consideration of therapy. Now attempt Activity 7.1.

Activity 7.1a   Treatments for pain
Activity 7.1b   Types of analgesic

Allow 30 minutes

Now would be an ideal time to study the activities entitled 'Treatments for pain', and 'Types of analgesic', which you will find on the DVD associated with this book. The first sequence includes shots of a surgical intervention to lower pain as well as interviews with the surgeon and other therapists. In Activity 7.1a Dr Ordman makes a reference to 'tricyclics'. These were first developed as a class of antidepressant medication. The use of such medication for the treatment of pain is described in the text. The second sequence illustrates some treatments for pain with animations and looks at aspirin, lignocaine and morphine in terms of their actions on the nervous system; interactive questions allow you to test your understanding of the effects of these chemicals.

If you are unable to complete these activities now, continue with the rest of the chapter and return to them as soon as you can.

Summary of Chapter 7

7.1   The term 'analgesia' refers to a procedure that lowers pain and a chemical that does this is an 'analgesic'.

7.2   Aspirin blocks the release of prostaglandins and thereby acts as an analgesic.

7.3 Lignocaine blocks the transmission of action potentials, by blocking ion channels in the cell membrane of the axon.

7.4 Opiates target synapses in the CNS that would, under natural conditions, employ opioids and thereby opiates act as analgesics.

7.5 Antidepressants can have a role in the treatment of pain.

7.6 Transcutaneous electrical nerve stimulation (TENS) activates neurons that have large-diameter axons and thereby tends to 'close the gate' in the nociceptive pathway and reduce pain.

7.7 Psychological interventions attempt to change the patient's cognition, so as to 'feel in control' and 'experience hope'. This appears to trigger a descending pathway that 'closes the gate'.

Learning outcomes for Chapter 7

After studying this chapter and its associated activities, you should be able to:

LO 7.1 Define and use, or recognise definitions and applications of, each of the terms printed in **bold** in the text. (Questions 7.1 and 7.2)

LO 7.2 Identify some means of treating pain and explain their mode of action. (Questions 7.1 and 7.2 and DVD Activities 7.1a and 7.1b)

LO 7.3 Show some links between psychological interventions and their possible biological bases. (Questions 7.1 and 7.2 and DVD Activities 7.1a and 7.1b)

If you are studying this book as part of an Open University course, you should also be able to:

LO 7.4 Perform an internet search using Boolean logic and keywords connected with pain, summarise aspects of the article and write a reference to it using a standard referencing convention. (Questions in Activity C1 in the *Companion*)

LO 7.5 Reflect on your strategy for organising information and consider ways to improve it. (Questions in Activity C2 in the *Companion*)

Self-assessment questions for Chapter 7

You also had the opportunity to demonstrate LOs 7.2 and 7.3 by answering questions in DVD Activity 7.1b.

Question 7.1 (LOs 7.1, 7.2 and 7.3)

Match the type of analgesic substance (1–3) to the mode of action (a–c).

(1) aspirin

(2) lignocaine

(3) opiate

(a) inhibits the synaptic effect of nociceptive neurons in the spinal cord

(b) blocks the release of prostaglandins

(c) blocks ion channels in the cell membrane of axons.

Question 7.2 (LOs 7.1, 7.2 and 7.3)

Successful psychological interventions for pain might be expected to increase the release of which of the following:

(i)   opiates

(ii) opioids

(iii) prostaglandins?

8 PLACEBO EFFECTS

The term **placebo effect** is difficult to define. As one (albeit imperfect) attempt at definition, it refers to the beneficial result of an intervention that has no *intrinsic* capacity to affect an outcome (Melzack and Wall, 1988). Nonetheless, the intervention exhibits a capacity to do so as a result of *the context in which it occurs*. For example, if the patient believes that it will help, even a sugar pill might have some effect in reducing pain. Of course, by virtue of its *intrinsic* chemical content, sugar has no known analgesic effect. Rather, the context in which it is taken is the significant factor.

In the scenarios introducing this book, the case of Natasha and her receipt of morphine was discussed. It was noted that, in an early research study, occasionally the morphine was omitted from the injection and yet the patients still derived some pain relief simply from the act of injection itself (Beecher, 1959). In such cases, the context was one of having experienced the injection of morphine earlier and obtaining pain relief from it. Replacing the morphine with a neutral substance keeps the context of the 'treatment' identical.

So-called 'neutral chemicals', e.g. a sugar pill, that are ingested or injected are a well-known example of a trigger to the placebo effect (Melzack and Wall, 1988). Coloured tablets have a greater potency than white tablets. Injections of neutral chemicals are more effective than swallowing the same substance. There is a surgical placebo: simply opening someone up, as though for therapeutic surgery, can sometimes have a beneficial effect (Cobb et al., 1959).

8.1 Explaining the placebo effect

How do psychologists explain the placebo effect? What kind of process underlies it? Evidence suggests the existence of, at least, two processes (Stewart-Williams and Podd, 2004), as follows.

8.1.1 Classical conditioning

The term 'conditioning' has entered popular culture, where it is sometimes used almost as a term of derision, as in 'they have simply been conditioned to act that way'. It suggests mindless 'robots' acting blindly. Such an image does not do justice to the phenomenon, which is ubiquitous across species and serves a very important adaptive role (Box 8.1).

Box 8.1   (Explanation) Pavlov and classical conditioning

Conditioning was first studied scientifically by the Russian physiologist Ivan Pavlov, in a famous experiment on salivation in dogs. Pavlov was interested in dogs' reactions to the presence of meat in the mouth. Meat triggers both salivation and the secretion of gastric juices by the stomach. Pavlov noted, quite incidentally, that a stimulus presented repeatedly with the meat (e.g. a person bringing the meat) would itself come to trigger salivation, even on occasions when the same person appeared but without the meat. These observations led to a formal scientific study.

Pavlov tried pairing the sound of a bell with the presentation of food a second or so later. After repeated paired presentations of the sound and food, even if the sound alone were presented, the dog would come to salivate to this. Prior to the pairing with food, the sound had no capacity to trigger salivation. After the pairing with food, the bell acquired the capacity to trigger salivation. This capacity was *conditional upon* the pairing with food, and hence arose the term 'conditioning'. See Figure 8.1.

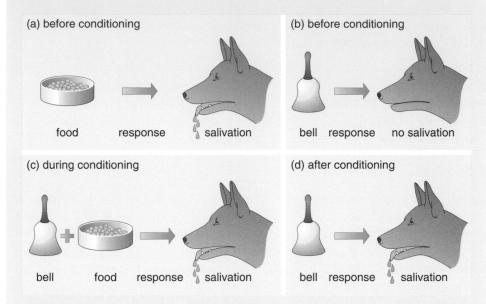

(a) before conditioning

food   response   salivation

(b) before conditioning

bell   response   no salivation

(c) during conditioning

bell   food   response   salivation

(d) after conditioning

bell   response   salivation

Figure 8.1　A schematic representation of the stages in classical conditioning.

Since this was the first type of conditioning to be studied scientifically, it became known as **classical conditioning** and is also termed 'Pavlovian conditioning'. It is easy to appreciate the adaptive value of classical conditioning when applied to a natural environment. For example, on hearing or seeing cues predictive of gaining food, an animal starts to secrete saliva and juices that aid digestion in the stomach. On contacting food, the animal is in an advantageous position to start the processes of feeding and digestion.

Suppose that following conditioning in Pavlov's experiment, the bell is repeatedly presented but without being accompanied by food. The bell will gradually lose its capacity to trigger salivation, a process known as **extinction**.

Analgesia is not so easy to understand as salivation but, none the less, the principle of classical conditioning can be applied to it.

◆ Applying the principle, what might normally be paired with the morphine?

◆ The sight and sound of the doctor, the sight and feel of the injection.

◆ How could the principle of classical conditioning be applied to the analgesia that can occur when the morphine is occasionally omitted from an injection and instead a neutral substance is injected?

◆ There has been a series of arrivals of morphine in the body and thereby analgesia in association with the presentation (e.g. sight of a syringe). Therefore, the injection procedure itself, even when the morphine is omitted, can come to trigger some analgesia.

Indeed, rather as with Pavlov's dog and salivation to the bell, a history of association between an injection and pain relief triggers some 'placebo' analgesia when the morphine is omitted. Such a process explains a part of the placebo effect and this aspect is not confined to humans.

The next section describes another factor also underlying the placebo effect.

8.1.2 Conscious insight

As far as we know, humans are unique amongst species in that they have a sophisticated language that mediates understanding of the world in terms of what causes what. With the help of both spoken and internal ('silent') language, humans form conscious expectations of what is going on (Figure 8.2). A conscious expectation can be formed by verbal suggestion from a therapist or from the patient's own interpretation of the situation. One such concerns pain relief. A patient in a medical context has a certain expectation of a favourable outcome and normally has a degree of trust in the expertise of medical staff to facilitate this. Thus, instructing someone that a pill will reduce pain can have just that effect, even though the pill might have no intrinsic pain-related properties, i.e. it is a pure placebo.

Expectations and hopes are features of the conscious mind, e.g. expectations of better things to come. Alas, people can equally create expectations of hopelessness and thereby sometimes exacerbate their pains.

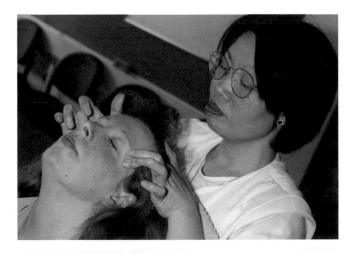

Figure 8.2 What sort of expectations does a patient bring to an interaction of this kind? (Photo: Mike Levers/Open University)

8.2   The psychobiology of the placebo effect

Some might claim that the placebo effect exemplifies 'mind over matter'. If this is taken to mean that psychological factors mediate the effect, then it would seem to be correct. However, caution is needed in the use of the expression 'mind over matter', since it could go against the well-formulated assumptions of psychobiology. It might suggest that there is a psychological factor ('mind') that is divorced from biology ('matter') and yet can still mysteriously affect matter. The perspective adopted here is that psychological factors are, simultaneously, *also* brain, and thereby biological, factors.

A similar logic applies to the lay use of the term 'psychosomatic'. The term consists of the roots 'psyche', meaning mind, and 'soma', meaning body. This suggests that something arises in the mind but none the less can still affect the body. If the term is taken to mean a psyche that is not in the body can still affect the body, it is misleading. However, if it refers to psychological factors that are *simultaneously* represented in the brain and can thereby affect various sites in the body, then it is entirely in keeping with psychobiology.

8.2.1   Brain imaging of the placebo effect

Brain imaging can link the psychology of the placebo to its biological roots and reveal the placebo effect in action. For example, in a study carried out in Vancouver, patients suffering from Parkinson's disease were presented with placebo medicine (de la Fuente-Fernández et al., 2002). Parkinson's disease arises from a loss of neurons that release the neurotransmitter dopamine in a region of the brain. Therapy consists of giving a drug to try to boost the limited levels of dopamine release that still remain. Imaging techniques showed increased dopamine release in the affected brain region as a result of the drug but also following placebo treatment. So, although the placebo *treatment* is non-specific, the *effect* here was specific.

Another study looked at patients suffering from irritable bowel syndrome (IBS), a disorder of chronic abdominal pain and disrupted patterns of defecation (Lieberman et al., 2004). Placebo treatment caused:

1   increased activity in a region of cortex outside the pain matrix

2   decreased activity in the pain matrix

3   decreased reported pain.

Evidence points to regions of cortex at the front of the brain as being a site of a cognitive process underlying analgesia, which exerts its effect by means shown in Figure 3.4a.

8.3   Implications of the placebo effect

The placebo effect is important for the development of new treatments. Suppose that a company claims that a drug is useful for treating pain. How do they know that any effect is not 'simply' a placebo effect? In order to persuade, for example, a government health ministry to adopt the new drug, researchers would need to show that its effect is *better than placebo*. So, one group of patients is treated with the drug and another with placebo and investigators see whether the first group shows a better result than the second.

◆ Is there another consideration in the design of the study?

◆ The patients should not know into which group they have been allocated.

◆ Why is this?

◆ Simply knowing that you are in the treatment group might in itself influence the outcome via the placebo effect. The drug might have no effect above the placebo level.

This is termed a **blind study**. Ideally, neither should the therapists who are treating and assessing the patients know to which group a particular patient has been allocated; this is termed a **double-blind study**. Otherwise, if the therapists have some vested interest in the success of the therapy, they might unwittingly treat the patients differently or interpret the outcomes in ways that support their favoured theory.

Summary of Chapter 8

8.1   The term 'placebo effect' describes something that has no intrinsic capacity to cause a particular effect but which shows some capacity by virtue of the context in which it occurs.

8.2   The placebo effect arises from both classical conditioning and from the patient's conscious insight into the situation.

8.3   Brain imaging reveals placebo treatments to have a measurable effect in reducing activity in the brain's pain matrix.

8.4   Tests for a new drug require a double-blind trial so that any efficacy above the placebo level can be identified.

Learning outcomes for Chapter 8

After studying this chapter and its associated activities, you should be able to:

LO 8.1   Define and use, or recognise definitions and applications of, each of the terms printed in **bold** in the text. (Question 8.1)

LO 8.2   Using pain as an example, describe which processes are thought to underlie the placebo effect. (Question 8.1)

LO 8.3   Describe some of the implications of the placebo effect for research into treating pain, including development of new treatments. (Question 8.1)

Self-assessment questions for Chapter 8

Question 8.1 (LOs 8.1, 8.2 and 8.3)

Consider the injection procedure associated with repeated morphine injection and the placebo effect derived from this. According to the principles of classical conditioning, what would weaken the placebo effect?

9   FINAL WORD

Chapters 1–8 have described some explanations of pain and also some of the various puzzles, paradoxes and anomalies of pain. For example, pain is a major health problem causing intense and unremitting misery to millions of people worldwide, yet carers and the medical sciences have only the subjective evidence of the sufferer as a measure of pain. Everything else is a proxy measure.

The chapters presented evidence that, in spite of the existence of specialised nociceptive neurons with sensory endings throughout most regions of the body, there is not a simple one-to-one link between tissue damage and pain. There can be intense pain with little evidence of tissue damage but, under other circumstances, there can be serious tissue damage with little pain.

The chapters have shown where a *psychobiological perspective* involves calling upon diverse sources of information. These include a consideration of early evolution and 'the human zoo', knowledge of the nervous system, but also understanding of the patient's lifetime experiences and the social-cultural context within which he or she lives. How pain and its relief fit to the conscious expectations and beliefs of the patient is vital in understanding pain and the associated reactions, as exemplified by such things as cultural differences in pain reaction and the placebo effect.

You might suppose that, from adaptive considerations, a straightforward link between tissue damage and pain would make sense. In these terms, how is the complexity of pain to be explained? The phenomenon of wind-up was explained in terms of a general nervous system property of plasticity but such insights can explain only a little of the complexity of pain.

Pain is essentially personal – a subjective phenomenon – but one obviously related to the brain, behaviour and sociocultural context. A reminder of the subjectivity of pain and taking a cross-cultural perspective suggests caution: outward expressions of pain do not necessarily map simply to subjective distress. Despite the sophistication of the science of pain, the most reliable measure is surely still the patient's own report. So, comparing *between individuals*, it is difficult, if not impossible, to answer the question – is one person's pain as bad as another's? However, comparing *within a given individual*, it is possible to get sensible answers to the question – is a person's pain better or worse following an intervention such as a drug or cognitive-behavioural therapy? Simply ask the patient.

At the heart of the search for explanations of pain, attention is drawn to the broader puzzle of how to relate the brain and the conscious mind. As the book draws to an end, it is time to make this issue more explicit, which this final chapter now does.

9.1   A challenging puzzle

When researchers examine what makes up a body, including the brain, they find only components that are described as 'physical', such as water, vitamins and blood cells. This is a world of *material objects* described in *physical* terms.

For example, the membrane that surrounds each cell is composed of such substances as fats and proteins. Atoms form molecules. Ions move across membranes, as in the action potential.

When investigators say that the cause of a pain is 'nociceptive', as in toothache, they can describe this in *physical* terms. There is the swelling at the root of the tooth and this causes electrical changes at nociceptive endings. Electrical events, termed action potentials, travel along the axons of nociceptive neurons and then reach the brain. All this is well understood in terms of physical and chemical events. Similarly, the evidence points to activity within particular populations of billions of neurons in the brain as being the *physical basis of pain*. When people react to this physical activity (associated with 'pain'), by means of the somatic nervous system, there is triggering of sets of skeletal muscles in such a way as to try to lower pain. Via the autonomic nervous system, there is an increased rate and intensity of the heart beat. So far, so good, in that we have traced a sequence of causes from sensory input through the brain and out to the muscles, and so to behaviour and physiological reactions.

At this point, if not much earlier, you might wish to protest that a cunning sleight of hand has been performed before your eyes. We would only request that you direct any protest not to the authors alone but to the failings of two thousand or so years of intellectual effort by philosophers, and later by psychologists and brain scientists. You might have followed the logic but find that something profoundly important is missing. It was said that activity of neurons is the *physical basis of pain* but this raises a series of closely related, perplexing and fundamental questions:

- In such an account of physical events, how and where does the awful conscious raw *feel* of pain appear?
- Why does it *feel* like anything *at all* to have this pattern of electrical activity in the brain?
- What is it about a *particular population* of neurons that means that it yields the conscious sensation specifically of *pain* when it is active?

These are all reflections of the same fundamental question: how does inanimate physical matter give rise to subjective conscious awareness? Alas, it will not be answered here or, in the foreseeable future, anywhere else. No one knows. In exactly the same way, no one knows why activity of a different set of neurons is experienced as conscious joy. So, if this book had been about romantic love or sexual desire, a pattern of activity of neurons in the brain (at a different location from the pain matrix) would have been described with the argument that this is its physical basis.

What we have just described is known as the **hard problem of consciousness**, so-called because no one can see any way of solving it. The hard problem is associated with a set of closely related questions, such as – why is only a limited amount of the information processed by the brain associated with conscious awareness? How are only *certain patterns* of activity by the brain associated with conscious awareness? Again, we can only plead that we do not know. However, even living with the mystery, we hope that you can still appreciate the relevance of examining the nature of the conscious mind and its contents to understanding pain.

By contrast, there are a number of so-called 'easy problems' of consciousness. These are of the kind, for example, that asks which particular brain regions are involved with which particular aspect of consciousness. The present book has posed a number of such (relatively!) 'easy problems'.

9.2 Relevance of the meaning of 'psychological' and 'psychogenic'

Related to the hard problem, the book has employed the term 'psychological' and noted that events described in these terms correspond to events in the physical brain. Consider a psychological intervention for relieving pain, such as distraction. According to a psychobiological perspective, any effect of this treatment will be manifest in changes in the activity of the brain.

A similar logic applies to the use of the term 'psychogenic'. Parminder was said to be in pain as a result of being jilted. Clearly, the trigger to her pain cannot be described in quite such straightforward terms as for a rotten tooth or ulcer, much as Parminder might, in her less charitable moments, be tempted to do so. Parminder looks at the 'jilting letter' and light from the words on the page falls on her retina at the back of the eye. The light sets up electrical activity in neurons and action potentials are conveyed to her brain. The brain deciphers the meaning of the words and then the awful significance of the message hits home. This is psychogenic pain. However, the phenomenon is also physical, since the account just given inevitably described a sequence of electrical events in the nervous system.

9.3 Practical implications

There are some important practical day-to-day implications of taking a psychobiological approach to pain. The broad dissemination of such an understanding of pain is likely to affect how pain patients view their own pain. The inclusion of psychological factors could be seen as a theoretical rationale for some empowerment of the patient.

People are occasionally reluctant to admit that psychological factors, such as stress or moods, play a role in pain. They fear that the pain will be dismissed as 'just psychological' and thereby not real (Keefe et al., 2005). To some people, psychological or psychiatric accounts seem to suggest personal weakness and failing, that is to say, lack of will and motivation, at the basis of the disorder. The patient can easily feel stigmatised. Similarly, a person might be reluctant to consider a psychological intervention on the grounds that this might cast doubt on the 'real' physical nature of their pain. In a study of non-cardiac chest pain, some patients withdrew their cooperation on being told of a psychological dimension and treatment option (Looper and Kirmayer, 2002). Anything to allay such patients' fears is welcome and a psychobiological understanding could help.

Physicians are sometimes impatient with people who report pain for which there is no obvious noxious stimulus evident. Indeed, the unflattering term 'litigation neurosis' has occasionally been applied to these patients. A psychobiological perspective allows such pain to be assessed as possibly being just as real as that associated with noxious stimuli. Brain imaging techniques offer a possible way of distinguishing pain of whatever origin from malingering. A person faking pain would be unlikely to be able to produce the patterns of brain activation associated with real pain.

On getting to the end of the book, you have covered a very large territory, ranging from electrons through neurons and brains to consciousness and social interactions between people. Who knows what secrets of pain and its possible treatment remain to be revealed within this network of interacting layers? We cannot anticipate what new drug or psychological treatment might lie in wait. However, we can promise that the explanation of how any such new treatment works will be greatly aided by your insights into the contemporary understanding of pain.

Summary of Chapter 9

9.1 Understanding how consciousness arises from inanimate matter is known as the 'hard problem of consciousness'.

9.2 A psychobiological perspective on pain can help to dispel myths and prejudice concerning psychological treatments.

Learning outcomes for Chapter 9

After studying this chapter and its associated activities, you should be able to:

LO 9.1 Define and use, or recognise definitions and applications of, each of the terms printed in **bold** in the text. (Questions 9.1 and 9.2)

LO 9.2 Describe what the 'hard problem of consciousness' is and what is so hard about it. (Questions 9.1 and 9.2)

LO 9.3 Argue the case for the value of a psychobiological perspective for treating pain. (Question 9.2)

Self-assessment questions for Chapter 9

Question 9.1 (LOs 9.1 and 9.2)

In asking which of the following questions (a) to (c), does one confront the hard problem of consciousness?

(a) Where do agonists and antagonists to the transmission of nociceptive signals act?

(b) What is the effect on pain of surgical damage to part of the brain's cortex?

(c) Why is activity of particular brain regions associated with an unpleasant conscious feeling?

Question 9.2 (LOs 9.1, 9.2 and 9.3)

Suppose that a patient is suspicious of psychological therapy, pleading that it feels as if the therapist is saying that the pain is 'all in the patient's mind'. Armed with the insights of a psychobiological perspective, what might you say to allay such fears?

ANSWERS AND COMMENTS

Answers to self-assessment questions

Question 1.1

According to a psychobiological approach, the mind encompasses all the information-processing carried out by the brain – or, put another way, the brain *is* the biological basis of the mind. Pain is simultaneously an experience of the conscious mind and a product of the body: a physical disturbance in a particular part of the body is communicated to the brain and this information is processed, understood and, as a feature of the mind, is interpreted as pain.

Question 1.2

(a) The presence of an infection is open to objective measurement, independent of the sufferer's conscious mind; for example, the causative bacteria or viruses may be identified by laboratory tests.

(b) Researchers can pose a wide range of challenges and make an objective measurement of the ability to reach out and grasp an object.

By contrast, the central focus of a study of pain must be the patient's own subjective report. The pain cannot be independently verified and there are ethical and practical barriers to triggering pain for experimental study.

Question 1.3

A commonly used proxy measure for self-managed pain is the number of painkillers, such as aspirin and paracetamol, sold per head of population. However, people vary a lot in whether or not they take painkillers and in how many tablets they take for different sorts of pain. Estimates of the extent of 'minor' pains based on such sales have a high degree of uncertainty.

Question 2.1

For a given physical disturbance, pain can be made worse by the patient putting a catastrophic interpretation on it or if the patient suffers from anxiety or depression.

Question 2.2

Imaging techniques have shown that some of the regions of the brain that are triggered into relatively high activity at times of nociceptive pain (the 'pain matrix') are also activated during psychogenic pain.

Question 3.1

(a) Nociceptive pain warns of tissue damage or potential tissue damage. Taking action to reduce it protects the body and thereby aids survival and reproduction chances. (b) A threat to a social bond is the trigger to psychogenic pain. Such bonds are vital to survival and reproduction in a social group-living species such as humans.

Question 3.2

(i) and (ii) are both proxy and objective measures (heart-rate does not directly measure pain); (iii) is clearly a subjective measure.

Question 3.3

The evidence includes the fact that certain regions of the brain are particularly active at times when noxious stimuli are applied to the body and, correspondingly, conscious reports indicate pain. Pain can be lowered by surgical removal of parts of the brain. When hypnosis for pain is successful, changes in the activity of specific regions of the brain are seen.

Question 4.1

As an example of homeostasis, (a) it is important for survival that body water level is maintained nearly constant and (b) indeed, the optimal body water level is defended. Dehydration is a reduction in water level below the norm. Information on this is *fed-back* to the brain to trigger drinking. Drinking corrects ('negates') the deficit.

Question 4.2

In each case, a disturbance to the body tending to move something away from the optimum is resisted. Action is triggered that serves to counteract the disturbance.

Question 4.3

(a) Epinephrine is like a key and its receptor is like a lock. (b) At times of emergency, epinephrine is secreted in relatively large amounts. This helps to prepare the body for 'fight or flight' by, for example, accelerating heart rate. This action can aid survival in threatening situations.

Question 5.1

A break in this location would result in a loss of sensation from the part of the body below the break and a loss of control over the muscles of the body below this level.

Question 5.2

(i) Neurons 1 and 4. (ii) The branch of the axon of neuron 2 associated with the label 'to brain'.

Question 5.3

The presynaptic neuron releases the neurotransmitter glutamate and the postsynaptic neuron (i.e. where receptors are occupied by neurotransmitter) has receptors that can bind glutamate specifically.

Question 5.4

A decrease in the frequency of action potentials produced in neuron 3, because the agonist would have the same effect as neurotransmitter released at the inhibitory synapse made by neuron 2.

Question 5.5

(i) The triggering of pain; (ii) increase in rate of heart beat.

Question 6.1

(a) (iii) Interneuron. (b) An increase in pain. Activity in the two axons described excites the S cell and causes the release of enkephalins. These tend to block transmission, i.e. 'closing the gate'. An antagonist to them would block their effect, i.e. to 'open the gate'.

Question 6.2

Arrow 2 in Figure 3.4b represents the influence of positivity in decreasing pain.

Question 6.3

(i) and (iii) characterise wind-up.

Question 6.4

Pain reported as appearing to originate in a part of the body which no longer exists and where the pain has got worse over time.

Question 6.5

(i) Excitatory.

Question 7.1

1b, 2c, 3a.

Question 7.2

(ii) Opioids.

Question 8.1

Repeated injection of a neutral substance without the accompanying morphine, i.e. extinction.

Question 9.1

Part (c).

Question 9.2

When a psychological technique for alleviating pain works, it is possible to see objective measures of a reduction in pain, in terms of brain activity. Thereby, the reluctant patient can be reassured that the therapy is affecting body *and* mind simultaneously.

Comments on the Activities

Activity 5.1

Figure 5.21 shows the completed graph.

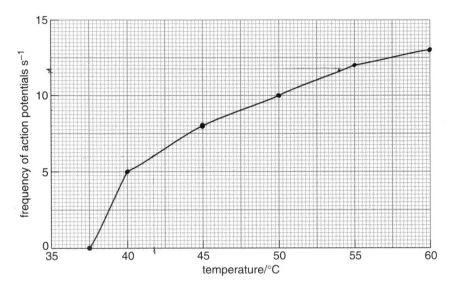

Figure 5.21 Line-graph showing action potential frequency as a function of temperature.

REFERENCES AND FURTHER READING

References

ABPI (Association of the British Pharmaceutical Industry)(2007) [online]. Available from: http://www.abpi.org.uk/publications/publication_details/ targetPain/tp1_intro.asp (Accessed March 2007)

Andersson, G. B. J. (1999) 'Epidemiological features of chronic low-back pain', *The Lancet*, vol. 354, pp. 581–585.

Beecher, H. K. (1946) 'Pain in men wounded in battle', *Annals of Surgery*, vol. 123, pp. 96–105.

Beecher, H. K. (1959) *Measurement of Subjective Responses*, New York, Oxford University Press.

Brennan, P. L., Schutte, K. K. and Moos, R. H. (2005) 'Pain and use of alcohol to manage pain: prevalence and 3-year outcomes among older problem and non-problem drinkers', *Addiction*, vol. 100, pp. 777–786.

Callister, L. C., Seminic, S. and Foster, J. C. (1999) 'Cultural and spiritual meanings of childbirth: Orthodox Jewish and Mormon women', *Journal of Holistic Nursing*, vol. 17, pp. 280–294.

Caraceni, A., Cheville, A. and Portenoy, R. K. (2000) 'Pain management: Pharmacological and nonpharmacological treatments', in Massie, M. J. (ed.), *Pain: What Psychiatrists Need to Know*, Washington, American Psychiatric Press, pp. 23–88.

Cheville, A., Caraceni, A. and Portenoy, R. K. (2000) 'Pain: definition and assessment', in Massie, M. J. (ed.), *Pain: What Psychiatrists Need to Know*, Washington, American Psychiatric Press, pp. 1–22.

Clark, R. W. (1980) *Freud – The Man and the Cause*, New York, Random House.

Cobb, L. A., Thomas, G. I., Dillard, D. H., Merendino, K. A. and Bruce, R. A. (1959) 'An evaluation of internal-mammary-artery ligation by a double-blind technic', *New England Journal of Medicine*, vol. 260, pp. 1115–1118.

Craig, A. D. (2003) 'Pain mechanisms: Labelled lines versus convergence in central processing', *Annual Review of Neuroscience*, vol. 26, pp. 1–30.

de la Fuente-Fernández, R., Phillips, A. G., Zamburlini, M., Sossi, V., Calne, D. B., Ruth, T. J. and Stoessl, A. J. (2002) 'Dopamine release in human ventral striatum and expectation of reward', *Behavioural Brain Research*, vol. 136, pp. 359–363.

Dubuisson, D. and Melzack, R. (1976) 'Classification of clinical pain descriptions by multiple group discriminant analysis', *Experimental Neurology*, vol. 51, pp. 480–487.

Edwards, C. L., Fillingham, R. B. and Keefe, F. (2001) 'Race, ethnicity and pain', *Pain*, vol. 94, pp. 133–137.

Eisenberger, N. I., Lieberman, M. D. and Williams, K. D. (2003) 'Does rejection hurt? An fMRI study of social exclusion', *Science*, vol. 302, pp. 290–292.

Eysenck, M. (ed.) (1998) *Psychology: An Integrated Approach*, Addison Wesley Longman Limited.

Frank, A. O. (2002) 'Back pain', *Rheumatology*, vol. 41, 1069–1070.

Gatchel, R. J. and Weisberg, J. N. (2000) *Personality Characteristics of Patients with Pain*. Washington, American Psychological Association.

Halliday, T. R. and Davey, G. C. B. (eds) (2007) *Water and Health in an Overcrowded World*, Oxford, Oxford University Press.

Harrison, A. (1991) 'Childbirth in Kuwait: the experiences of three groups of Arab mothers', *Journal of Pain and Symptom Management*, vol. 6, pp. 466–475.

Hobara, M. (2005) 'Beliefs about appropriate pain behavior: cross-cultural and sex differences between Japanese and Euro-Americans', *European Journal of Pain*, vol. 9, pp. 389–393.

IASP (2007) *IASP Pain Terminology* [online]. Available from: http://www. iasp-pain.org/AM/Template.cfm?Section=Pain_Definitions&Template=/CM/ HTMLDisplay.cfm&ContentID=1728#Pain (Accessed March 2007)

Keefe, F. J., Abernethy, A. P. and Campbell, L. C. (2005) 'Psychological approaches to understanding and treating disease-related pain', *Annual Review of Psychology*, vol. 56, pp. 601–630.

Lieberman, M. D., Jarcho, J. M., Berman, S., Naliboff, B. D., Suyenobu, B. Y., Mandelkern, M. and Mayer, E. A. (2004) 'The neural correlates of placebo effects: a disruption account', *Neuroimage*, vol. 22, pp. 447–455.

Looper, K. J. and Kirmayer, L. J. (2002) 'Behavioral medicine approaches to somatoform disorders', *Journal of Consulting and Clinical Psychology*, vol. 70, pp. 810–827.

MacDonald, G. and Leary, M. R. (2005) 'Why does social exclusion hurt? The relationship between social and physical pain', *Psychological Bulletin*, vol. 131, pp. 202–223.

McLachlan, H. and Waldenström, U. (2005) 'Childbirth experiences in Australia of women born in Turkey, Vietnam and Australia', *Birth*, vol. 32, pp. 272–282.

Melzack, R. (1988) 'IASP President's address: The tragedy of needless pain: a call for social action', in Dubner, R., Gebhart, G. F. and Bond, M. R. (eds), *Proceedings of the Vth World Congress on Pain*, Amsterdam, Elsevier Science Publishers, pp. 1–11.

Melzack, R. and Wall, P. D. (1988) *The Challenge of Pain*, London, Penguin Books.

Midgley, C. A. (ed.) (2008) *Chronic Obstructive Pulmonary Disease: A Forgotten Killer*, Oxford, Oxford University Press, in press.

Mounce, K. (2002) 'Back pain', *Rheumatology*, vol. 41, pp. 1–5.

Müller, T., Mannel, M., Murck, H. and Rahlfs, V. W. (2004) 'Treatment of somatoform disorders with St. John's Wort: A randomized, double-blind and placebo-controlled trial', *Psychosomatic Medicine*, vol. 66, pp. 538–547.

Patterson, D. R. (2004) 'Treating pain with hypnosis', *Current Directions in Psychological Science*, vol. 13, pp. 252–255.

Phillips, J. B. (ed.) (2008) *Trauma, Repair and Recovery*, Oxford, Oxford University Press, in press.

Phillips, J. M. and Gatchel, R. J. (2000) 'Extraversion-introversion and chronic pain', in Gatchel, R. J. and Weisberg, J. N. (eds), *Personality Characteristics of Patients with Pain*, Washington, American Psychological Association, pp 181–202.

Roth, R. S. (2000) 'Psychogenic models of chronic pain: A selective review and critique', in Massie, M. J. (ed.), *Pain: What Psychiatrists Need to Know*, Washington, American Psychiatric Press, pp. 89–131.

Russo, E. (1998) 'Cannabis for migraine treatment: the once and future prescription? An historical and scientific review', *Pain*, vol. 76, pp. 3–8.

Salomons, T. V., Johnstone, T., Backonja, M. M. and Davidson, R. J. (2004) 'Perceived controllability modulates the neural responses to pain', *Journal of Neuroscience*, vol. 24, pp. 7199–7203.

Stewart-Williams, S. and Podd, J. (2004) 'The placebo effect: Dissolving the expectancy versus conditioning debate', *Psychological Bulletin*, vol. 130, pp. 324–340.

Sufka, K. and Turner, D. (2005) 'An evolutionary account of chronic pain: Integrating the natural method in evolutionary psychology', *Philosophical Psychology*, vol. 18, pp. 243–257.

Sullivan, M. D. (2000) 'DSM-IV Pain disorder: a case against the diagnosis', *International Review of Psychiatry*, vol. 12, pp. 91–98.

Wade, J. B. and Price, D. D. (2000) 'Nonpathological factors in chronic pain: Implications for assessment and treatment', in Gatchel, R. J. and Weisberg, J. N. (eds), *Personality Characteristics of Patients with Pain*, Washington, American Psychological Association, pp. 89–107.

Ware, M. A., Doyle, C. R., Woods, R., Lynch, M. E. and Clark, A. J. (2003) 'Cannabis use for chronic non-cancer pain: results of a prospective survey', *Pain*, vol. 102, pp. 211–216.

Wong, D. L., Hockenberry-Eaton, M., Wilson, D., Winkelstein, M. L. and Schwartz, P. (2001) *Wong's Essentials of Pediatric Nursing* (6th edn), St. Louis, M. Mosby.

WHO (2002) *Revised Global Burden of Disease (GBD) 2002 Estimates* [online]. Available from: http://www.who.int/healthinfo/bodgbd2002revised/en/ (Accessed March 2007)

WHO (2004) *Headache disorders* [online]. Available from: http://www. iasp-pain.org/AM/Template.cfm?Section=Pain_Definitions&Template=/CM/ HTMLDisplay.cfm&ContentID=1728#Pain (Accessed March 2007)

Further reading

Aydede, M. (2006) *Pain: New Essays on its Nature and the Methodology of its Study*, Massachusetts, Bradford Books. [Covers the more philosophical and theoretical issues surrounding pain and its study.]

Melzack, R. and Wall, P. D. (1996) *The Challenge of Pain*, London, Penguin Books. [A classic text that is still relevant.]

Moerman, D. E. (2002) *Meaning, Medicine and the 'Placebo Effect' (Cambridge Studies in Medical Anthropology)*, Cambridge, Cambridge University Press.

Thorn, B. E. (2004) *Cognitive Therapy for Chronic Pain*, New York, Guilford Press. [Details the use of cognitive therapy in treating pain.]

Wall, P. D. (1999) *The Science of Suffering (Maps of the Mind)*, London, Weidenfeld and Nicholson. [Another perspective on pain by one of the two architects of gate theory.]

Winterowd, C., Beck, A. T. and Gruener, D. (2003) *Cognitive Therapy with Chronic Pain Patients*, New York, Springer Publishing Co. Inc. [Another perspective on the use of cognitive therapy in treating pain.]

Useful websites, maintained by the OU Library through the ROUTES system:

http://www.jr2.ox.ac.uk/bandolier/booth/painpag/ (a valuable resource for investigating many aspects of pain)

http://www.pain.com/ (a comprehensive guide to various sources of information on pain)

http://en.wikipedia.org/wiki/Pain_and_nociception (some good leads to various aspects of pain)

http://www.nlm.nih.gov/medlineplus/pain.html (the site of an official US government medical body)

http://www.iasp-pain.org//AM/Template.cfm?Section=Home (the website of the International Association for the Study of Pain)

http://www.elsevier.com/wps/find/journaldescription.cws_home/506083/ description#description (for the journal *Pain*, one of the major publication outlets of original research on pain)

http://www.britishpainsociety.org/ (the website of the British Pain Society, the professional UK body for the study and treatment of pain)

http://www.wellcome.ac.uk/en/pain/index.html (the pain section of the website of the Wellcome Trust, a distinguished UK body that supports medical research)

http://www.painrelieffoundation.org.uk/ (The Pain Relief Foundation, a UK charity dedicated to trying to alleviate pain)

ACKNOWLEDGEMENTS

Grateful acknowledgement is made to the following sources for permission to reproduce material in this book.

Figures

Figure 1.1: Natalie Behring/Panos Pictures; Figure 1.2: Frank, A. O. (2002) 'Recurrent tenosynovitis in Sweets syndrome', *Rheumatology*, vol. 41. British Society for Rheumatology; Figure 1.3: Mark Henley/Panos Pictures;

Figure 2.1: Jim Varney/Science Photo Library; Figure 2.2: Francoise Sauze/ Science Photo Library;

Figure 3.1: Wong, D. L. and Hockenberry-Eaton, M. J. (2001) *Wong's Essentials of Pediatric Nursing*, 6th edn, Mosby; Figure 3.2: ©2004 Credit:Topham Picturepoint; Figure 3.5: © Porzellan Manufaktur Staffelstein GmbH & Co. KG.;

Figure 4.1b: Eysenck, M. (ed.) (1998) *Psychology: An Integrated Approach*, Addison Wesley Longman Limited;

Figure 5.2c: Paul Gabbott; Figures 5.8 and 5.12: Toates, F. (2001) *Biological Psychology: An Integrative Approach*, Pearson Education Ltd; Figure 5.18a: CC Studio/Science Photo Library; Figure 5.18b: Wellcome Dept. of Cognitive Neurology/Science Photo Library;

Figure 6.6: SedatAral/Rex Features; Figure 6.10: Photolibrary.Com (Australia);

Figure 7.2: Eye Ubiquitous/Rex Features; Figure 7.3: BSIP, MENDIL/Science Photo Library.

Tables

Table 3.1: Melzack, R. and Wall, D. (1988) *The Challenge of Pain*, Penguin Books Ltd.

INDEX

Entries and page numbers in **bold type** refer to key words which are printed in **bold** in the text. Indexed information on pages indicated by *italics* is carried mainly or wholly in a figure or a table.

A

action potential 47–50, 96, 100, *102*
  analgesic effect on *78*, 79
  energy requirements 57
  and pressure applied 64, 65, *66*
  at synapses 51–2, *54*, *55*
acute pain 7
adaptive value 15–17, 26, 28, 43, 59, 99
  analgesia and 84–5
  of plasticity 70–1
adrenalin *see* epinephrine
affect 26
affective dimension of pain *18*, 26, 68
agonists 55, 62, 77, 79, 100
alcohol 11, 81
Alzheimer's disease 23
anaesthetics 23
analgesia 77, 84–5
  classical conditioning and 90–1
analgesics 19, **77**–9, 80
  numbers prescribed 29, 99, 100
  types of 85, *86*
angina 3, 20
ANS (autonomic nervous system) 59, 60
antagonists 55, 75, 77, *78*
antidepressants 80, 85
anxiety 12, 20, 21, 99
arthritic pain 3, *4*, 17, *18*, 21
aspirin *78*, 79, 85, *86*, 99
atoms 44, 45–6
autonomic nervous system (ANS) 59, 60
axon 32, *33*, *39*, 40, *41*, 62, 100
  descending axon *67*, 68, 75
  diameter of 64, 65, 67, 68
  movement of action potential along *48*
axon terminal *41*, 48, 51, *52*

B

back pain 4, 12, *18*
  psychological factors and 8–9
battery 46
binding site *34*
biology 2, 77
biopsychosocial 2
blind study 93
blood vessel *33*, 59, *60*
body systems 31–2
body temperature regulation 32, 34, 35, 38, 59, 100
brain *39*
  cerebral hemispheres 56–7
  coordination role 60
  and interpretation of pain 10–11, 31
  nociceptive information pathway *63*, 68–9
  nutrients 55–6
  role in pain 22–5, 29, 100
  see also **mind**
brain cells *37*
brain damage 23, 58
brain imaging 12, 13, **57**, 73, *74*, 97–8, 99
  placebo effect 92
brain surgery 23, 58, 64, 100

C

cancer pain 8, 10, 17, *18*, 21
cannabis 80–1
cardiac muscle 59
'catastrophising thoughts' 12, 84, 99
cell membrane 32, *33*, *34*
  potential difference across 46, 47
'cell-to-cell communication' 34
cells 32–4
central nervous system (CNS) 39
cerebral arteries 55, *56*
cerebral hemispheres 56–7

chemical compound 44
chronic pain 7, 12
  evolutionary trade-off 17
  and plasticity 70
  surgery for 82, 85
circulatory system 31
classical conditioning 89, **90**, 91, 93, 101
CNS (central nervous system) 39
coca leaves *80*
cocaine 80
cognition 25–6
cognitive-behavioural therapy (CBT) 26, **83**–4
cognitive processes 25–6
conscious insight 91
conscious mind 2, 25–8, 91, 100
consciousness, hard problem of 96, 98, 101
controllability of pain 82, 83
coordination, nervous system and 60
corpus callosum *56*
cortex *56*, **57**, *63*, 68, 92
cortisol *36*, *37*
cultural factors in pain 80–1, 95

D

dehydration 38, 100
dental surgery 79
depression 4, 7, 12, 20, 21
  antidepressants 80, 85
descending axon *67*, 68, 75
developed countries, pain statistics 3, 4
developing countries, pain statistics 3, 4
disc disease pain *18*
distraction techniques 12, 26, 27
'disturbance to the body' 1, 2, 7, 9, 31, 100
dogs, salivation 89–90
dopamine 92

double-blind study 93

drug addiction 81

drugs
cultural, social and legal dimensions 80–1
see also **analgesics;** antidepressants; *individual drugs*

E

electric current 46

electrons 33, **44**, 45

elements 44

emotional pain *see* depression; **psychogenic pain;** psychological pain

empathy 9, 10, *11*, 16, 74

endocrine glands *36*

endocrine system 36–7

endogenous 55

endorphins 55

enkephalin receptors *67, 68, 79*

enkephalins *67, 68, 81*, 101

epinephrine 16, *36, 37, 38, 59, 62*, 100

ethnicity 22

evaluative dimension *18*

evolution
and pain 15–17, 95
and pain relief 84–5

evolutionary trade-off 17

excitatory synapse 53, *54, 58, 68, 69, 70*, 76, 101

experimental study of pain 2, 17, *18, 19*

extinction 90, 101

extracellular fluid *33*, 46

extroverts 20

F

'flight, fright or fight hormone' *37, 59*, 100

fluid environment of the body 32, 34

frequency of action potentials 49, *50, 102*

G

GABA (gamma-aminobutyric acid) 53

gate theory 66–7, *68, 69*, 82, 101

gender, and pain 22

global statistics, on pain *4*

glutamate 53, *62, 66, 75*, 100

H

hard problem of consciousness 96, 98, 101

headaches 3, *4*

heart rate 19, 29, *37*, 59, 60, 100

helplessness, feelings of 83, 84

heroin 11, 79, 80

homeostasis 34, 35, 37, 38, 59, 100

hormones 16, **36,** *37*, 45

hypnosis 12, 23, **84,** 100

I

incidence of pain *4*

industrial injuries disablement benefit *4*

infectious and parasitic diseases, objective measurement 6, 99

inhibitory synapse 53, *54*, 58, 76

injections 12, 89, 90–1, 93, 101

injuries *4, 18*, 21

insulin *36*

interneurons 40, *41*, **42,** 66, 75, 101

interpersonal violence *4*

intracellular fluid *33*, 46

introverts 20

invalidity benefit *4*

ion 45, 46, 47

ion channels 47, 79, 87

irritable bowel syndrome 92

K

kidneys *36*, 37

L

labour pain *18*, 22

legislation, and drug taking 80, 81

leprosy 43

life expectancy 17

lignocaine *78, 79*, 85, 86

litigation neurosis 97

lock-and-key interaction 33, *34*, 36, 37, 38, *51*, 100

lumen 59, *60*

M

macromolecules 45

malingering 98

mastectomy, phantom sensations 71

meditation 12

menstrual pain *18*

mind 2, 6, 12, 22, 91, 99
and consciousness 25–8, 95–7, 100

molecules 33, **44**–5

morphine 11, 12, 55, 79, 85, 89, 90–1, 93, 101

motor neuron 40, *41*, **42,** 50, 75

muscles
loss of control 61, 100
movement of 42, 50
pain 10, 15
skeletal muscle 58, *59*, 60
smooth muscle *33*, 59, 60

Mycobacterium leprae 43

N

negative affect 26

negative feedback 35, 37, 38, 100

nerves 23, 24, 32, *39*, 40, 62, 100

nervous system 31, 39–61, 100

neurogenic pain 68–9, 70, 72

neuron 32, *33*, 62, 100
and body temperature regulation 35
mode of action 44–50
role in pain 43–4
role in reflexes 42–3
types of 40, *41*, 42, 75
see also **axon;** nociceptive neuron; **sensory neuron; synapses**

neurotransmitter 51–3, *55, 62, 75*, 100
antagonists targeting 77, *78*
release of 70

neutral chemicals 89, 91, 101

neutrons 44

nociception 10

nociceptive ending 40, *41*, 43, 48, *63*, 65, 79

nociceptive information pathway *63*, 64–9

nociceptive neuron 43, 50, 62, *63, 78*, 95
within the spinal cord 66–7, 87
threshold of excitation 64–6

nociceptive pain 10, 12, 13, 20, 99
    adaptive value of 28, 99
    related to psychogenic pain 73–4
    role of neurons and 40, 42
    triggers to *24, 25*
non-cardiac chest pain 84, 97
noxious stimuli 10
    defence against 44
    and magnitude of pain 63, 100
    and pain 21–2, 23
nucleus (atom) 44, 45, *47*
nucleus (cell) 32, *33*
nutrients for the brain 55–6

O

obesity 16
objective measurement 3, 17, 19, 29, 99, 100
occupational injuries 4, *5*
oestrogen *36*
opiates *78*, **79**, 80, 81, 84, 85, 86, 87
opioid agonists 79
opioids 55, 68, 79, 81, 87, 101
opium 80, 81
organs 32
osteoarthritis *4*
ovaries *36*

P

pain 1
    adaptive value of 15–17
    anomalies of 69–73
    describing and classifying 7–13, 99
    examples of 1, 8
    interacting factors underlying 20–1
    measuring 2–5, 6, 99
    nature of 17–20
    periphery of the body and *63*, 64–6
    psychobiological approach to 2, 6, 99
    role of brain in 22–5, 29, 100
    role of neurons in 43–4
    spinal cord and 66–8
    and stimuli 21–2, 23
    treatment 77–87, 95, 101
    types of 9–10
pain clinic 19

pain matrix 12, *24*, 25, 57, *63*
    damage to 58
    and pain controllability 82, 83
pain rating scale 17, 19, 29, 100
'pain-stress cycle' 83
painkillers *see* **analgesics**
pancreas *36*
'paradox of pain' 10, 13, 21, 69–73
Parkinson's disease 92
pathway 58, *59*, *63*
Pavlovian conditioning 89–91, 93, 101
peripheral nervous system 39
    nociceptive information pathway *63*, 64–6
phantom limb 23, 71, *72*
phantom pain 71–2, 76, 101
physiology 31, 39
pituitary gland *36*, 37
placebo effect 12, **89**, 95
    explaining 89–91
    implications of 92–3
    psychobiology of 92
plasticity 69–71, 75, 95
positive outlook 12, *24*, 25, 26, 75, 84, 101
postsynaptic neuron 51, 52, 53, *55*, 62, 75, 100
potential difference 46–7, 48
presynaptic neuron 51, 52, 53, *55*, 62, 75, 100
prevalence of pain 4
prostaglandins 65, *66*, 79, 87
proteins 45
protons 44
proxy measures 3, 6, 29, 95, 99, 100
psychobiological approach 2, 6, 11, 25, 77, 95, 99
    and the placebo effect 92
    practical implications 97–8, 101
psychogenic pain 11, 12, 13, 20, 75, 97, 99, 101
    adaptive value of 28, 99
    related to nociceptive pain 73–4
    triggers to *24, 25*
psychogenic stimuli 11
psychological pain 7–8, 8–9, 10–11, 12, 58
    see also depression

psychological therapies 12, 82–5, 87
    suspicions of 97, 98, 101
psychology 2, 77
psychosomatic 92

R

receptor 34, 36, *37*, 62, 100
    action at synapses 51–2, *53*, 55
    enkephalin receptors *67*, 68, 79
referred pain 72–3
reflex 42–3, 58
religious factors 22, 68, 95
respiratory system 31
resting potential *47*

S

S cell *67*, 68, 75, 101
St John's Wort 80
salivation 89–90
self-efficacy 83, 84
self-inflicted injuries *4*
self-managed pain 6, 99
sensation, loss of 61, 100
sensory dimension *18*, 20
sensory neuron 40, *41*, 75
    threshold of excitation 64–5
    warm-sensitive 48–50
    see also nociceptive neuron
sensory route *24, 25*
serotonin 80
severe disability allowance *4*
side-effects 77
signalling molecule 33, 34, 36, 45–6
skeletal muscle 58, *59*, 60
smooth muscle *33*, 59, *60*
social bonds 16
social rejection 10, 12, 20, 25, *74*, 99
social security benefits *4*
sociocultural factors 22, 95
    drugs 80–1
sodium chloride 45
somatic nervous system (SNS) 58, 60
somatisation 20
spinal cord 23–4, *39*, *41*, 61, 100
    injured *4*
    nociceptive information pathway *63*, 66–8

stimuli *see* **noxious stimuli; psychogenic stimuli**

stoicism 22, *68*

stress 17, 21, 25, 83

stroke 56

subjective experience 2, 3, 12, 17, 19, 29, 95, 99, 100

substance P 66, *67*, 68

suprarenal glands *36*, *37*, 59

surgery
    brain surgery 23, 58, 64, 100
    chronic pain 82, 85
    dental surgery 79

surgical placebo 89

synapses 51–3, 58, 62, 100
    excitation and inhibition at 53–4, 68, 76, 101
    manipulating 54–5
    plasticity 69, *70*
    in the spinal cord *67*

T

temperature
    and action potential frequency *49*, *50*, *102*
    see also body temperature regulation

temporal dimension 7, *18*, 20

TENS machine 81, *82*, 85

testes *36*

testosterone *36*

thalamus *63*, 66, 68

threshold of excitation 64–6, 67

threshold of pain 22

thyroid gland *36*

thyroxin *36*

tissue damage 10, 15, 23, 99
    and nociceptive neuron activity 64, 65, 66, 95

tissues 32

toothache 10, 12, *18*, 96

tract 43, *62*, 100

traffic accidents *4*, 5

transcutaneous electrical nerve stimulation (TENS) **81**–2, 84, 85

transmission cells 66, *67*, 68, 71, *72*, *73*

tricyclics 85

U

unconscious processing 27

urbanisation, sources of pain 5, 16

V

vasopressin *36*, 37

voltage 46, 47, 48

W

warm-sensitive neuron 48–50

water
    molecule *45*
    sodium chloride dissolving in 45

wind-up 70–1, 75, 95, 101

Wong-Baker Faces pain scale *19*

World Health Organization, pain statistics 3, *4*

Z

zero affect 26

zoos 16